INJURY PREVENTION IN CHILDREN

INJURY PREVENTION IN CHILDREN

A Primer for Students and Practitioners

by

David H. Stone

Professor of Paediatric Epidemiology,
The University of Glasgow

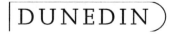

Published by
Dunedin Academic Press Ltd
Hudson House
8 Albany Street
Edinburgh EH1 3QB
Scotland
www.dunedinacademicpress.co.uk

ISBN 978 1 906716 25 7

British Library Cataloguing in Publication data
A catalogue record for this book is available from the British Library

Typeset by Makar Publishing Production
Printed in Great Britain by CPI Antony Rowe

FSC
www.fsc.org
MIX
Paper from
responsible sources
FSC® C013604

Contents

Acknowledgements

Many people gave me the encouragement and practical help that proved so necessary to propel this book from conception to completion. In particular, I am grateful to the University of Glasgow for granting me a period of sabbatical leave that gave me the essential time and space to undertake the task; to my secretary, Rita Dobbs, who 'held the fort' for me back in the office while the project was underway; to my PEACH Unit colleagues, Krista Kleinberg and Mhairi Campbell, whose eagle eyes greatly enhanced the quality of the text; to Michael Hayes, of the Child Accident Prevention Trust, who offered much detailed and perceptive expert advice on the content; and to the countless students and colleagues who have, over many years, reinforced my conviction that child injury prevention is, and will remain, one of the most exciting and productive branches of global public health.

Preface

Purpose and scope of the book

Injury prevention remains a relatively neglected branch of public health. As it rises up the political and professional agenda, as it is bound to do given the increasing emphasis on an evidence-based and data-driven approach, the need for high-quality training materials will inevitably grow. This book is an introductory text that summarises the key principles of injury prevention and how these may be translated most effectively into practice and policy-making. Its perspective is a public health one, and the writing style informal, jargon-light and accessible yet authoritative.

The focus of the book is on children, defined loosely as people up to school-leaving age – anywhere between 14 and 19 years old. The World Health Organization, taking its cue from the United Nations Convention on the Rights of the Child, suggests that birth to 18 years is the appropriate range, although, in the absence of an internationally accepted definition of childhood, some degree of flexibility is required. This book has sought to follow that precedent. As for injury, most types are included, whether intentional (violence and self-harm) or unintentional ('accidental'). Unfortunately, some topics have received short shrift either through lack of space or because the interested reader is well served by alternative texts. One of these is travel safety, a term that should encompass injury prevention despite its strong emphasis on infectious diseases. Another that receives minimal attention is occupational safety as it generally refers to the adult working population (although child labour, both legal and illegal, remains all too common in many parts of the world). Also excluded are most forms of sporting injuries, psychological trauma that is unrelated to physical injury, and adverse effects or complications of medical interventions.

Who is this book for?

The majority of readers will probably not be entering injury prevention full time but will wish to undertake injury prevention or safety promotion training modules for the purpose of accreditation or promotion. Potential readers include medical and nursing undergraduate/postgraduate students, public health trainees, community safety professionals, local authority officials, research students, civil servants, politicians and journalists. No prior knowledge of the subject matter is needed, but some familiarity with the basic concepts of epidemiology and public health will be helpful to the reader.

The structure of the book and how to use it

The book comprises three sections. The first outlines the principles of injury prevention that underpin all policy-making and practice in the field. The second applies the principles in a way that demonstrates how the main players can translate them into action. The third and final section looks to the future and identifies some of the key challenges that are likely to face all those concerned with injury prevention in the next few decades. Each section is composed of four chapters. Each chapter starts with a statement of learning objectives and ends with a summary. Some key learning points and practice nuggets are interspersed throughout the book.

Effective injury prevention is a difficult and challenging activity. Many aspects of it are controversial and sometimes divisive. Throughout the book, key disputes are presented in the form of 'heated debates' that seek to steer readers through the various arguments in a manner that will enable them to decide for themselves whether or not they agree with the writer's conclusion.

The book ends with a list of key messages to which readers may refer from time to time to refresh their knowledge without necessarily having to delve in detail into the text. At the end of the References there is also a list of useful websites on injury prevention for readers wishing further information.

Glossary of terms

Attempted suicide (or parasuicide)
'Attempted suicide' and 'parasuicide' are terms that refer to an unsuccessful attempt to take one's own life intentionally.

Audit
Audit is used to assess the extent to which an intervention meets a standard that is regarded as good practice.

Burden of injury
The burden of injury on the population is the impact of injury measured by financial cost, mortality, morbidity or other indicators. It is often quantified in terms of two related indicators: quality-adjusted life–years (QALYs) and disability-adjusted life–years (DALYs).

Child abuse
Child abuse is all forms of physical and emotional ill-treatment, sexual abuse, neglect, and exploitation that result in actual or potential harm to the child's health, development or dignity. To that may be added fabricated or induced illness.

Child maltreatment
Child maltreatment is an act or failure to act by a parent, care-taker or other person that results in physical abuse, neglect, medical neglect, sexual abuse, emotional abuse, or an act or failure to act that presents an imminent risk of serious harm to a child.

Collective violence
Collective violence is the instrumental use of violence by people who identify themselves as members of a group – whether this group is transitory or has a more permanent identity – against another group or set of individuals, in order to achieve political, economic or social objectives.

Critical appraisal
Critical appraisal is the process of systematically assessing research reports to judge their trustworthiness, value and relevance in a particular context.

Deliberate self-harm

Deliberate self-harm refers to any damaging activity that individuals deliberately inflict upon themselves, including cutting, 'overdosing' (self-poisoning), hitting, burning or scalding, pulling hair, picking or scratching the skin, self-asphyxiation, ingesting toxic substances and fracturing bones.

Effectiveness

Effectiveness is the extent to which an intervention has been shown to work in practice.

Efficacy

Efficacy is the extent to which an intervention has been shown to work in ideal or experimental conditions.

Ethics

Ethics refers to the rules or standards governing the conduct of a person or of the members of a profession.

Epidemiology

Epidemiology is the study of the distribution (incidence and prevalence) and determinants (aetiology) of health and disease in human populations.

Evaluation

Evaluation simply means 'to determine the value of', although it is commonly used to describe a research or audit method that compares a process or outcome with a predetermined objective or standard, or with a comparable control group.

Evidence-based public health

Evidence-based public health policy and practice comprise a triangulation that incorporates an assessment of scientific evidence, the judgement of the professional, and the perspective of the target population.

Hazard

A hazard is an object, substance, activity, circumstance or situation that can potentially cause adverse effects, such as a threat to life or health. When vulnerable individuals or populations or populations come into contact with a hazard, they are exposed to risk.

Hazard and risk

Hazard and risk are interrelated concepts that describe the dangers posed by environmental factors to humans. They are not, however, synonyms.

Injury

Injury occurs when a rapid transfer of energy – or the withdrawal of a life-sustaining element such as oxygen or heat – from the environment to a human being results in tissue damage.

Injury control
Injury control embraces activities that both prevent the occurrence of injury and seek to ameliorate its consequences (such as death or disability) either through preventive or harm-reduction approaches. The latter are designed to limit the degree of tissue damage, adverse health effects (including death), disability and costs following upon injury.

Injury incidence
The incidence of injury is the number of new cases arising in a defined population over a specified time period.

Injury prevalence
The prevalence of injury is the number of cases existing in a defined population at a specified point in time.

Injury prevention
Injury prevention is used to denote:
- ❑ the avoidance of the event leading to the injury (*primary prevention*);
- ❑ the avoidance or amelioration of the injury when an event occurs (*secondary prevention*);
- ❑ the avoidance of death, disability and other adverse consequences through the provision of adequate care and rehabilitation (*tertiary prevention*).

Policy
A policy (sometimes called a strategy or plan) is a written document that provides the basis for action to be taken jointly by the government and its non-governmental partners.

Public health
Public health is the science and art of preventing disease, prolonging life and promoting health through the organised efforts of society.

Premature mortality due to injury
Premature mortality is computed in various ways, the most common being the number of potential years of life lost through injury (the average life expectancy of the population minus the average life expectancy of injury victims).

Proportional mortality of injury
Proportional mortality is the relative contribution that injury makes to total mortality.

Risk
Risk is the likelihood that a hazard will actually cause its potential adverse effects, together with a measure of the effect. It is expressed, either quantitatively or qualitatively, as a probability of future harm occurring as the result of human exposure to one or more hazards.

Risk assessment

Risk assessment is the process of identifying and documenting actual or perceived risks to human safety to allow further evaluation and appropriate responses.

Safety promotion

Safety promotion refers to the range of measures, activities and policies that seek to reduce the frequency, severity and adverse consequences of injuries in the population. These measures are designed to reinforce those characteristics of people and communities which enhance the subjective feeling of being protected from the risk of injury from whatever source.

Screening

Screening is a process of identifying apparently healthy people who may be at increased risk of a disease or condition. They can then be offered information, further tests and appropriate treatment to reduce their risk and/or any complications arising from the disease or condition.

Suicide

Suicide is the act of taking one's own life intentionally.

Surveillance

Surveillance (a term sometimes used synonymously with monitoring) is the systematic, continuous and purposeful collection, analysis and reporting of data on a health topic with a view to the detection, reporting and, where appropriate, response to deviations from a predetermined norm.

Trauma

Trauma is a synonym for physical injury, although it may also be used to describe either acute or chronic emotional, psychological, familial or social disruption.

Violence

Violence is the intentional use of physical force or power, threatened or actual, against oneself, another person or a group or community that results in injury, death, psychological harm, impaired development or deprivation.

SECTION 1

PRINCIPLES OF INJURY PREVENTION

Section 1 Overview

This section comprises four chapters and their summaries. These outline the principles of injury prevention that underpin all policy-making and practice in the field. The chapter titles are:

1. Introduction, concepts, definitions, history

2. Epidemiology and natural history of injury

3. Preventive approaches to injury

4. Implementation and evaluation.

CHAPTER 1

Introduction, concepts, definitions, history

Learning objectives

- To have a basic grasp of the nature of injury as a public health challenge
- To be able to define injury
- To understand the concepts of injury prevention and injury control
- To be able to classify injuries into their basic types
- To be aware of the key milestones in the history of injury prevention

Injury as a public health challenge

Injuries and violence are threats to health in every country and every community. Worldwide, more than five million people die each year as a result of some form of injury, and many more remain disabled for life. Given current trends, the global burden of injuries and violence is expected to rise considerably during the coming decades, particularly in low- and middle-income countries.

In terms of potential years of life lost, child injuries are one of the leading – and growing – global public health challenges. In 2002, over 700,000 children under the age of 15 died as a result of an injury. Indeed, injuries are the leading cause of death worldwide for children after their first birthday, although there is considerable variation between countries. The World Health Organization (WHO; Murray and Lopez, 1997a) predicts that injury will rise up the global league table of premature mortality (from ninth place to third), with road casualties especially becoming more burdensome. There is also high morbidity associated with childhood injuries: for every injured child who dies, several hundred are hospitalised with painful and disrupting injuries, and several thousand live on with varying degrees of discomfort, distress and disability. While a large proportion of these injuries are the result of road crashes, many (e.g. falls, burns and drownings) occur either in the home or in leisure environments.

Despite the growing numerical significance of this problem, injury has only recently come to be perceived as a public health problem that merits sustained attention. And even today, few countries have national policies, strategies or plans of action for injury and violence prevention. Nevertheless, despite the topic having been seriously neglected in the past, governments, professionals and public health agencies around the world have recently begun to recognise the huge toll of avoidable suffering and expenditure that injuries cause. Moreover, injury disproportionately affects vulnerable sectors of society such as children, older people and the disadvantaged, thereby contributing to health inequalities. The result is that injuries are slowly but surely rising up the public health policy agenda in many countries and regions.

The main contribution of the growing body of epidemiological research on injuries since the Second World War may be summed up in five words – *injuries are not random events*. They are predictable and avoidable, perhaps to a greater extent than most other causes of mortality and morbidity in the early part of the human life cycle. Over the past few decades, a formidable amount of research evidence has accumulated that is available to guide practitioners and policy-makers. Although more research is always required, the full implementation of the existing body of evidence could substantially reduce the incidence and impact of injury.

◀ LEARNING POINT ▶

Injuries are not random events. They are predictable and avoidable, perhaps to a greater extent than most other causes of mortality and morbidity in the early part of the human life cycle.

What is injury?

Language is important for human communication. Unless we share a common understanding of the meaning of words, confusion will abound. In the public health field, words have to be selected with great care as misunderstandings can have serious consequences for patients and the population we are trying to protect. Nowhere is this more apparent than in the field of injury prevention. Until relatively recently, the most popular terms used to describe an injury (usually of the unintentional type) in medical and lay circles respectively have been 'trauma' and 'accident'. Neither, however, is satisfactory.

Trauma is really just a synonym for physical injury – although it may also be used to describe either acute or chronic emotional, psychological, familial or social disruption. It is an unsatisfactory term in some ways as it conjures up an image of a serious casualty arriving at a hospital emergency department with a scrum of white-coated staff weighing in with drips and defibrillators in an attempt to resuscitate the hapless victim.

The fact is that most injuries do not present in this way. Hospital-based serious trauma care – medical or surgical – is a hugely important aspect of modern healthcare, but it deals with a small minority of all injuries. Moreover, in common parlance, the term 'trauma' is frequently understood to refer to psychological rather than physical disturbance, or to a kind of nebulous mixture of the two. Although 'injury' is far from perfect, it seems destined to remain the preferred term until someone comes up with a more satisfactory alternative.

HEATED DEBATE No. 1: Accident or injury?

The injury prevention community has steadfastly eschewed the term 'accident' while almost everyone else persists in its frequent use. The question is: does it matter?

An *accident* is an unintentional injury or, more precisely, the event or process leading to the injury. The term is rapidly becoming obsolete in the scientific and public health literature, where its use is regarded as nurturing archaic and potentially counterproductive notions of unpredictability, randomness and unavoidability. On the other hand, the substitution of 'injury' for 'accident' is often unsatisfactory as the former is an outcome while the latter is an event or series of events or a process.

'Accident' is such a problematic word that the *British Medical Journal* (Davis and Pless, 2001) took the controversial decision to banish it from its pages on the advice of injury researchers. The journal asserted that this was necessary to counter what they perceived as a residual attitude of fatalism to the phenomenon of injury. Their arguments may be paraphrased as follows. First, the concept of an accident excludes intentional injury despite the fact that intent is often difficult or impossible to establish. Second, the phrase 'accidents will happen' reflects a collective assumption that such events are random, unavoidable and unpredictable. We now know that this assumption is simply untrue. We can assert with confidence the opposite – that in many (perhaps most) cases, 'accidents will not happen' if appropriate action is taken based on an accumulating knowledge about risk factors, causes and effective countermeasures. Nevertheless, we should recognise that the general public and many professionals continue to use the term in a way that does not necessarily preclude prevention (Girasek, 1999).

Conclusion

If we accept the proposition that language is important in the communication of ideas, we must try to seek a resolution to this debate. Given that many professionals find the word 'accident' unacceptable, and that the general public is unfamiliar with the term 'trauma', that leaves us with only one remaining contender – 'injury'. Although far from perfect, as it refers to an outcome rather than a precursor event or process, it has become the common currency of the global injury prevention community. Without adopting an excessively dogmatic position, and recognising its inherent weaknesses, the term 'injury' appears to be the preferred option in most circumstances.

Injury occurs when a rapid transfer of energy – or the withdrawal of a life-sustaining element such as oxygen or heat – from the environment to a human being results in tissue damage. In common public health usage, the term 'injury' *excludes* psychological trauma (although that may be consequent upon physical injury) and food poisoning as well as certain other categories such as chronic exposure to chemicals, radiation, etc. Adverse effects of medical care (medical 'accidents') are also usually excluded form the definition of injury (although there are divergent views on this).

In its report on childhood injury, the WHO paraphrases the definition of injury offered by Baker *et al.* (1992):

> the physical damage that results when a human body is suddenly subjected to energy in amounts that exceed the threshold of physiological tolerance – or else the result of a lack of one or more vital elements, such as oxygen.

In other words, injury is caused when human tissue is damaged by acute exposure to energy, whether mechanical, thermal, electrical, chemical or ionising radiation. Sometimes, however, injuries result from the sudden lack of essential agents such as oxygen or heat.

LEARNING POINT

Injury occurs when a rapid transfer of energy – or the withdrawal of a life-sustaining element such as oxygen or heat – from the environment to a human being results in tissue damage.

● ●

Injury prevention and injury control

As described above, injury prevention is used to denote:

❑ the avoidance of the event leading to the injury (*primary prevention*);
❑ the avoidance or amelioration of the injury when an event occurs (*secondary prevention*);
❑ the avoidance of death, disability and other adverse consequences through the provision of adequate care and rehabilitation (*tertiary prevention*).

Because, arguably, only the first and, to a limited extent, the second of these represents true prevention, the term *injury control* has been coined to describe the entire range of such activities. The all-embracing nature of the term is useful, but it its disadvantage is that it may unwittingly promote a drift of policy and practice focus away from primary and secondary prevention towards acute trauma care and rehabilitation.

HEATED DEBATE No. 2:
Injury prevention, injury control or safety promotion?

Terminology evolves in response to changing knowledge, professional preference or mere fashion. The phrase 'injury prevention' remains widespread but has begun recently to be complemented or even supplanted by two alternative notions: 'injury control' and 'safety promotion'. It is entirely plausible that one of those latter terms will eventually dominate to the point where it becomes the norm. Which of these three phrases is preferable? There is no easy answer.

Injury prevention is a public health term that refers to the range of measures, activities and policies that seek to reduce the frequency, severity and adverse consequences of injuries in the population. Its philosophical premise is clear: injury should be avoided or, if it cannot be, its severity should be minimised.

The broader concept of *injury control* recognises that, even when injury cannot be avoided, much can be done to improve the prognosis of the victims. Injury control embraces activities that both prevent the occurrence of injury and seek to ameliorate its more serious consequences (such as death or disability) through either preventive or harm-reduction approaches. The latter are designed to limit the degree of tissue damage, adverse health effects (including death), disability and costs following upon injury. Its use has been strongly advocated by researchers who point to the impressive reductions in injury case fatality rates that have been achieved by high-quality healthcare, particularly as practised by regional trauma centres.

Both these ideas may seem straightforward enough, yet many public health professionals are abandoning them in favour of a third: *safety promotion*. This more recent development is due neither to chance nor to fashion but to a fundamental philosophical shift that, in turn, derives from similar trends occurring within the broader public health community.

Safety implies freedom or protection from those conditions that can cause injury or death to personnel, or damage to or loss of equipment or property. Safety is the reciprocal of risk (actual or perceived) or indeed of injury itself. Conceptually, safety lies at the positive end of the health–disease spectrum, whereas injury lies at the negative end. The term is also frequently used to denote either (or both) an individual or a collective sense of security, i.e. freedom from violent assault or other crime or fear of crime.

Safety may be defined as the condition of being protected from external hazards or freedom from danger, risk or injury. It may be regarded as the outcome of successful injury prevention in much the same way as health is a consequence of disease prevention (Pless and Hagel, 2005). The term also suggests a combination of both subjective and objective components that may or may not be present concurrently.

Safety promotion is a term that refers to the range of measures, activities and policies that seek to reduce the frequency, severity and adverse consequences of injuries in the population. These measures are designed to reinforce those characteristics of people and communities that enhance the subjective feeling of being protected from the risk of injury from whatever source. Safety promotion may therefore be regarded as a specific form of health promotion, an idea that grew out of health education and subsequently embraced a broader agenda including social marketing. Both health promotion and safety promotion are useful in focusing attention on what the sociologist Antonovsky (1996) has called *salutogenesis*, or processes that promote heath via the nurturing of human resilience and other protective factors. These *salutogenic* processes may be regarded as representing the mirror image of *pathogenic* processes. Because 'health promotion' is often used synonymously with 'health education', some may associate safety promotion with an excessively individualistic approach to injury prevention.

Conclusion

Injury prevention and safety promotion could be regarded as two sides of the same coin. The former derives from the traditional health protection or prevention paradigm that seeks to influence favourably the *pathogenesis* (disease-producing process) of a disease or disorder, while the latter is based on a more modern health promotion paradigm that seeks to influence favourably *salutogenesis* (health-producing process) in individuals and populations. Injury prevention is the narrowest of the three, while safety promotion is the most holistic. Although all three concepts are valid, the trend towards safety promotion seems likely to continue in the foreseeable future.

Classification of injuries

The term 'injury' conveys nothing about intent. Conventionally, injury is strictly categorised either as *unintentional* ('accidental') or *intentional* (deliberate self-harm, suicide or violence). These methods of classification have evolved over time in a somewhat inconsistent manner and have been variously based on the characteristics of people (victims), cause, place and time. A consensus is slowly developing around the need to use, where possible, a single classification system such the International Classification of Diseases Tenth Revision (ICD 10) and the International Classification of External Causes of Injury (ICECI). The former tends to focus on the injury itself, with limited information on its circumstances or mechanisms, while the latter attempts to remedy this deficiency by providing a more detailed description of each injury.

Severity of injury is important for three main reasons: to describe the clinical status and aid the prognosis of injured patients presenting to hospital; to offer a more accurate epidemiological picture of the burden of injury; and to control for confounding in research. A great deal of research effort has been invested in this topic, and several scales have been developed to measure injury severity. These are discussed in more detail in Chapter 2.

Unintentional and intentional injury

The strict dichotomy between unintentional and intentional injury is increasingly regarded as untenable since intent may be impossible to determine with certainty. It may make more sense to think of injuries as spanning a spectrum of intent from clearly unintentional at one end to clearly intentional at the other. There is a substantial grey area within which intent may best be described as 'unknown' or 'undetermined' and where the risk of misclassification is high. Nevertheless, an attempt to distinguish between the two categories is often necessary and useful for the purposes of reporting, research or prevention.

◀ LEARNING POINT ▶

The strict dichotomy between unintentional and intentional injury is increasingly regarded as untenable since intent may be impossible to determine with certainty.

Unintentional injuries are often subdivided by their causal mechanisms or circumstances, in other words how they occurred. Popular subcategories (described in more detail in Chapter 2) are

- ❏ road traffic injuries;
- ❏ falls;
- ❏ burns and scalds;
- ❏ drowning;
- ❏ fire and flames;

❑   poisonings;

❑   others.

Some classification methods utilise the *place* where the injuries occurred – roads, home, school, leisure/sport, workplace. Others are based on the *time* of occurrence – during either working or leisure time.

Intentional injuries may be subdivided according to the *people* involved in the event:

❑   deliberate self-harm (suicide, attempted suicide, parasuicide);

❑   interpersonal violence (homicide, intimate partner violence, sexual abuse, child abuse and neglect, elder abuse);

❑   collective violence (e.g. war, civil uprising, criminality, terrorism).

Suicide is the act of taking one's own life intentionally. *Attempted suicide* and *parasuicide* are terms that refer to the unsuccessful attempt to take one's own life intentionally.

Deliberate self-harm refers to any damaging activity that individuals deliberately inflict upon themselves, including cutting, 'overdosing' (self-poisoning), hitting, burning or scalding, pulling hair, picking or scratching the skin, self-asphyxiation, ingesting toxic substances and fracturing bones. Broader types of self-harm, such as drug and alcohol misuse, are usually excluded from this definition.

Violence is the *intentional* use of *physical* force or power, threatened or actual, against oneself, another person or a group or community that results in injury, death, psychological harm, impaired development or deprivation.

The WHO defines *child abuse* as:

> all forms of physical and emotional ill-treatment, sexual abuse, neglect, and exploitation that result in actual or potential harm to the child's health, development or dignity. (www.who.int/topics accessed 7 February 2011)

To this may be added fabricated or induced illness.

The US Administration for Children and Families (www.acf.hhs.gov/programs/cb/systems/ncands/ncands98/glossary/glossary.htm accessed 18 February 2011) has defined *child maltreatment* as:

> An act or failure to act by a parent, care-taker, or other person as defined under State law which results in physical abuse, neglect, medical neglect, sexual abuse, emotional abuse, or an act or failure to act which presents an imminent risk of serious harm to a child.

The ill-defined 'grey area' between intentional and unintentional injuries usually arises either because intent is unknown (e.g. when the victim's account is ambiguous or when there are no witnesses) or when the recording of intent is deliberately circumspect due to potential medicolegal repercussions (e.g. when child abuse is suspected). Sometimes deliberate injury is not recorded for cultural or religious reasons (e.g. in many countries, the recording of suicide in official records is often avoided by resorting to the term 'undetermined cause of death').

Brief history of injury prevention

We often think of injury prevention as a relatively recent development in the annals of public health, but this is only partially true. Injury prevention actually has ancient origins. One of the earliest pieces of safety legislation in human history is described in the Bible:

> When you build a new house, you shall make a parapet for your roof, that you may not bring the guilt of blood upon your house, if anyone should fall from it. (Deuteronomy 22:8)

Little is known about injury prevention in the Middle Ages. It is safe to assume that, given the generally appalling living and working conditions experienced by most people, especially children, at that time, attention to safety was minimal. In the late 18th and early 19th centuries, the German physician Johann Peter Frank offered what was probably the first comprehensive plan for public health including the promotion of safety awareness. An American First World War pilot, Hugh DeHaven, having survived a serious plane crash, set about studying the biomechanics of passive safety and recommended, based on his findings, the routine wearing of helmets and seat belts in aircraft and cars.

In the mid-20th century, another breakthrough occurred when Harvard epidemiologist John Gordon applied the host–agent–environment infectious disease paradigm to injury (Gordon, 1949), opening the way for multifaceted approaches to prevention. In 1961, James Gibson, a psychologist, conceptualised injury in terms of the transfer of energy from the environment to human tissue. This was elaborated by William Haddon (1999), a public health doctor and engineer, who is widely acknowledged as 'the father of modern injury prevention' through his systematic analysis of the numerous ways in which this energy transfer (or lack thereof) comes about. His brilliant rearticulation of Gordon's triad in terms of three temporal injury event phases – prior to, during and following an injury – has stood the test of time (see Chapter 3). His lasting legacy, however, is probably the foundation he laid for future generations of injury prevention professionals, working largely within the public health paradigm that he advocated, to build upon.

The publication of the landmark report *Injury in America* (Committee on Trauma Research, 1985) gave a further boost to the field and unlocked generous funding in that country for a range of initiatives including the establishment of new injury prevention centres and the adoption of a high-profile role in surveillance, research, networking and guidance by the Centers for Disease Control.

◄ LEARNING POINT ────────────────────────────────

William Haddon, a public health doctor and engineer, is widely acknowledged as 'the father of modern injury prevention' due to his systematic approach to the analysis of injury occurrence.
● ●

SUMMARY OF CHAPTER 1

Introduction, concepts, definitions, history

- ■ Injuries and violence are threats to health in every country and every community. Worldwide, more than five million people (of whom around 700,000 are children) die each year as a result of some form of injury, and many more remain disabled for life.

- ■ Injury has only recently come to be perceived as a public health problem that merits sustained attention. And even today, few countries have national policies, strategies or plans of action for injury and violence prevention, although that is changing.

- ■ Injuries are not random events. They are predictable and avoidable, perhaps to a greater extent than most other causes of mortality and morbidity. Although more research is always required, the full implementation of the existing body of evidence could substantially reduce the incidence and impact of injury.

- ■ The term 'accident' is becoming obsolete in the literature, where its use is regarded as nurturing archaic and counterproductive notions of unpredictability and unavoidability. On the other hand, the substitution of 'injury' for 'accident' is often unsatisfactory as the former is an outcome whereas the latter is an event or series of events, or a process.

- ■ The World Health Organization defines injury as follows: 'Injuries are caused by acute exposure to physical agents such as mechanical energy, heat, electricity, chemicals, and ionising radiation interacting with the body in amounts or at rates that exceed the threshold of human tolerance. In some cases (e.g. drowning and frostbite), injuries result from the sudden lack of essential agents such as oxygen or heat.'

- ■ The dichotomy between unintentional and intentional injury is increasingly regarded as untenable since intent may be impossible to determine with certainty. It may make more sense to think of injuries as spanning a spectrum of intent from clearly unintentional at one end to clearly intentional at the other. There is a substantial grey area within which intent may best be described as 'unknown' or 'undetermined' and where the risk of misclassification is high.

- ■ Injury prevention is referred to in the Bible. In the 18th and 19th centuries, the public health movement advocated safety promotion. In the 20th century, a Harvard epidemiologist, John Gordon, applied the host–agent–environment infectious disease paradigm to injury. Gibson's subsequent conceptualisation of injury in terms of the transfer of energy from the environment to human tissue led William Haddon to offer a systematic analysis of the numerous ways in which this energy transfer (or lack) comes about and might be counteracted.

CHAPTER 2

Epidemiology and natural history of injury

Learning objectives

- To understand in greater detail why childhood injury is so important
- To know the key elements of the epidemiological approach to injury
- To be aware, in outline, of how injury risk varies by the key variables of geography, gender, socio-economic status, time and developmental stage (age)
- To have a basic knowledge of the descriptive epidemiology and natural history of common types of unintentional childhood injury
- To have a basic knowledge of the descriptive epidemiology and natural history of common types of intentional childhood injury
- To be aware of the links between mental health and childhood injury

Why is childhood injury so important?

The public health importance of childhood injury derives from two factors – the nature of childhood and epidemiology. First, the international public health community has a particular responsibility to promote and protect the health of the most vulnerable in society. Children are a vulnerable group who are, to a large extent, dependent on adults to articulate their needs and to fulfil their requirements for health, well-being and safety. Second, in most 'developed' (high-income) countries, injuries are the largest single cause of death in children and young people (numerically comparable to malignancy), and a major cause of morbidity as reflected by hospitalisation, emergency department (ED) attendance, primary care visits and long-term disability.

◀LEARNING POINT

In most high-income countries, injuries are the largest single cause of death in children and young people (numerically comparable to malignancy), and a major cause of morbidity.

• •

In the UK, unintentional injury mortality (although not necessarily incidence) has declined over the past 20 years for reasons that are not entirely clear. Declining injury mortality may reflect various influences including diminishing exposure to environmental hazards and improved trauma care rather than declining incidence.

Nevertheless, specific injury prevention measures are assumed to have contributed to some of this trend. By contrast, intentional injury mortality (violence, suicide) has increased and may overtake unintentional injury rates within a few years.

━LEARNING POINT━

Declining injury mortality may reflect improved trauma care and survival rather than declining incidence, although specific injury prevention measures are assumed to have contributed to some of this trend.

Globally, about 10% of all deaths and five of the 25 leading causes of death (road casualties, self-inflicted trauma, violence, drownings and war) are due to injury (Murray and Lopez, 1997b). Injury-related injury mortality is expected to rise up the burden of disease league table in the coming decades, from around five million deaths to over eight million by 2030, and the number of disability-adjusted life–years (DALYs) attributable to injuries will far exceed those from cardiovascular or respiratory disease.

The financial costs of injury are enormous: the direct costs of injury to the National Health Service in the UK are around £2 billion per annum, with the global costs to society perhaps 10 times that figure. The costs of child injury care at accident and emergency departments in the UK in 2008 (Audit Commission/Healthcare Commission, 2007) have been estimated at £146 million annually.

Two related reports published by the World Health Organization (WHO) recently highlighted the continuing importance of unintentional injuries in children from a European (Sethi et al., 2008) and a world (Peden et al., 2008) perspective. Injury in children and young people is increasingly recognised as the outcome of exposure to a hazardous environment. In Europe, injuries were estimated to be the cause of 23% of all deaths and 19% of DALYs in the age group 0–19 years. These figures dwarf other environmental causes of the disease burden such as air pollution, lead exposure, and inadequate sanitation (Valent et al., 2004).

Epidemiological approach to injury

Injury prevention relies to a large extent on epidemiology for an understanding of the nature, causes and frequency of injury as well as for the development, implementation and evaluation of countermeasures. All concerned with injury prevention therefore need to acquire some understanding of this basic science of public health.

Epidemiology is defined as the study of the distribution (incidence and prevalence) and determinants (aetiology) of health and disease in human populations. It is thus the basic science of public health. Like other disorders, injury is a multifaceted phenomenon that is manifested in various ways that can be described and quantified epidemiologically using well-established indicators. Some of these relate to *mortality* and others to *morbidity* (non-fatal occurrences). Each of these indicators should be viewed in the context of the precursors (risk or causal factors) and sequelae (consequences such as suffering, disability and economic costs).

Epidemiology is defined as the study of the distribution (incidence and prevalence) and determinants (aetiology) of health and disease in human populations. It is the basic science of public health.

Epidemiologists seek to characterise any disease in the most comprehensive manner possible but may be seriously hindered by the lack of data. Nevertheless, some attempt to construct a complete picture of the impact of the disease on the population, based on a conceptual model, is a useful starting point. A helpful way to think of the epidemiology of any condition is to visualise an iceberg or pyramid (Figure 2.1) with mortality at the tip, hospitalisations in the middle and incidence, including premorbid or relatively non-serious conditions along with causal or risk factors, at the base.

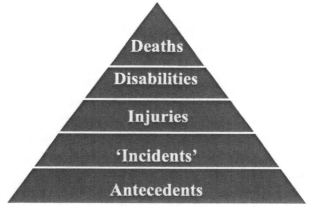

Figure 2.1 The injury pyramid.

There are other versions of the injury pyramid, including a simplified depiction on three levels – deaths, hospitalisations and healthcare presentations. Vyrostek *et al.* (2004) analysed injury data from the USA for the year 2001 and found a ratio of 10 hospitalisations and 178 presentations to each death. Analyses from other countries suggest a much steeper numerical gradient from the tip to the base of the pyramid.

Although the events or phenomena represented by the different levels of the injury pyramid are extremely heterogeneous, it is a powerful model for several reasons. First, it provides a graphic description of the relative proportions of injuries that present as different outcomes. Depending on the type of injury, these relative proportions vary, and the shape of the pyramid will reflect this. Second, it illustrates the relatively small number of more serious outcomes in the context of the totality of injury. And third, it shows how the various components of the pyramid relate to each other in time: by rotating the pyramid through 90 degrees, it becomes transformed into a sequence of successive and interrelated events or a 'natural history of injury' culminating in an outcome such as death, disability or resolution. This, in turn, may be used to stimulate thinking about prevention in the same way that the natural history of other diseases, such as cancer or cardiovascular disease, is the starting point for the development of interventions designed to improve their outcomes.

Once the natural history of any disease process is understood, it becomes possible to develop, implement and evaluate strategies to arrest or reverse the process and thereby reduce the number of victims and the burden of the condition on the population at risk.

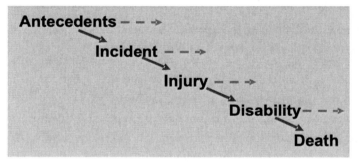

Figure 2.2 Natural history of injury.

Epidemiological measures of injury

Among the most widely used epidemiological measures of injury are incidence, prevalence, proportional mortality, premature mortality and burden of injury in the population.

The *incidence* of injury is the number of new cases arising in a defined population over a specified time period.

The *prevalence* of injury is the number of cases existing in a defined population at a specified point in time.

Proportional mortality is the relative contribution that injury makes to total mortality.

Premature mortality is computed in various ways, the most common being the number of potential years of life lost through injury (the average life expectancy of the population minus the average life expectancy of injury victims).

The burden of injury on the population is the impact of injury in an area measured by financial cost, mortality, morbidity or other indicators. It is most often quantified in terms of two related indicators – quality-adjusted life–years (QALYs) and disability-adjusted life years (DALYs) – which combine the burden due to both death and morbidity into one index. These allow for the comparison of the disease burden due to various risk factors or diseases and also make it possible to predict the possible impact of health interventions.

Of these two indicators, DALYs have become increasingly popular, with the encouragement of the WHO, around the world. This measure combines both mortality and morbidity, and takes account both of the years of life lost prematurely and those years of life lived but blighted by disability. It is calculated by adding the years of life lost (YLL) to the years of life lived with disability (YLD):

$$DALY = YLL + YLD$$

YLL is an aggregate of the ages of deaths of victims subtracted from the average life expectancy of that population, whereas YLD is calculated by applying a disability weighting to the aggregated years lived by victims from the injury event to death. The disability weightings are derived either from empirical research or from the judgement of an expert panel. One DALY is regarded as the equivalent of one healthy year of life lost.

Sources, range and quality of routine data

The reporting of *mortality statistics* is a statutory requirement in most countries of the world, although the quality varies widely. It is hugely tempting to accept injury mortality rates at their face value, but this would be a mistake. They are liable to contain numerous sources of error, including diagnostic inaccuracy, misclassification and bias, as these are almost inevitable in the production of such statistics. Because these are inconsistent between countries, international comparisons present major problems. Murray and Lopez (1997a) have pointed out that less than a third of the 50 million deaths in the world each year are medically certified. Moreover, mortality is the outcome of an interaction between incidence, severity and survival, each of which is influenced by a multiplicity of factors. Nevertheless, mortality data are attractive to epidemiologists because of their availability, lack of ambiguity (in the sense that death is rarely in dispute) and public health importance (in that they represent the most severe outcomes of a disorder).

Moving down a level in the injury pyramid, *hospitalisation statistics* are even more problematic. Not only are they subject to the same sources of error as mortality data, but they also suffer from the added disadvantage of being dependent to a large extent on the availability and uptake of hospital beds. To add to the confusion, hospital admission policies may vary widely for the same condition, and this will distort the data patterns. Thus, a low hospitalisation rate for injury may reflect a low level of bed provision, or a tendency not to admit injured patients, rather than a low incidence of injury. And the way in which hospitalisation data are coded diagnostically varies widely. In the case of injury, the specification of the circumstances of the injury is more important than the diagnosis for preventive purposes, and this information is rarely available from routine hospitalisation data.

At the base of the pyramid, large numbers of injuries present to the health services in ways that are not captured at all by routine statistics. Injuries to children may be self-treated or treated by parents or carers, or by community practitioners such as nurses, family doctors or teachers. Only some of these incidents will be recorded, and those that are may not be easily accessible. A reasonable and widespread assumption is that most severe injuries will be treated initially in hospital EDs (Emergency Department). Even if that were true, data from EDs are extremely patchy. Ideally, *all* EDs would record and report such information, but this is rarely undertaken (see the discussion on injury surveillance in Chapter 3). An even more fundamental gap is the virtually universal absence of injury incidence data apart from the limited information collected intermittently by some population surveys.

Measuring injury severity

Because of their numerical predominance, analysing data on non-fatal injuries is essential to try to understand the epidemiology and causes of injury in the population. Some of the challenges that this presents to the epidemiologist have been outlined above. Arguably, the greatest challenge of all lies in describing injury in terms of one of its most important characteristics – severity.

Clinicians working in trauma care have long regarded an assessment of severity – the degree to which an injury threatens survival or quality of life – as crucial as a guide to good clinical care and as a prognostic tool. Several clinical injury severity scores have been created with this in mind. These are based on the analysis of large numbers of injured patients in terms of their observed case fatality rates, and they have proved clinically extremely useful in the care of moderately or severely injured patients. The Abbreviated Injury Scale (AIS) is an anatomically based injury description system that scores an injury from 1 (minor) to 6 (virtually unsurvivable). The Injury Severity Score (ISS) is the summation of the squares of the highest AIS scores in three body areas. Both the AIS and ISS are popular with trauma researchers who analyse registry data, but they have not been extensively used epidemiologically (Cryer, 2006).

A six-point injury scoring method designed for children, the Pediatric Trauma Score (PTS), has also shown promise clinically but remains underutilised by epidemiologists. One reason for this is that the PTS, like the AIS and ISS, is often unsuitable for common forms of child injury such as drowning. A second is that it is difficult to use these severity scores to derive severity-specific rates in defined populations due to numerator–denominator mismatch (Alexandrescu *et al.*, 2009).

Why is severity important in public health terms? Consider the average family. All of its members will suffer at least one injury in the course of a year. Some of these will be trivial bumps, scrapes and bruises, while others may be potentially life-threatening. Indeed, injury is a completely normal part of growing up and of life itself. Because injury is such a universal human experience, we need to distinguish between injury that is significant from a preventive perspective and injury that is not. Setting a threshold of severity above which we record injury is one way of achieving this.

In many cases, the injury diagnosis that is recorded in routine health records (other than trauma registries) will convey almost nothing whatsoever about severity. Exceptions include bone fractures, at least some of which (e.g. skull or long bone fractures) may be assumed to be severe enough to require acute hospital care and may be used as a proxy for severity. Length of hospital stay has been used as a proxy for severity but is unsatisfactory as there may be social or medical reasons, unrelated to the injury, that cause a period of hospitalisation to be prolonged. Another epidemiological approach to measuring injury severity is the attempted 'translation' of injury diagnoses recorded by International Classification of Diseases Ninth Revision (ICD 9) into an ISS (MacKenzie *et al.*, 1989; Osler *et al.*, 1996; Cryer 2006).

Road safety is one area where the routine recording and reporting of severity has long been attempted, with only partial success. The UK classification of road casualties, for example, into fatal, serious and slight injuries is highly problematic as these categories, although reasonably well defined, are adhered to inconsistently by individual police officers at the scene of a crash. The result is that the accuracy and reliability of casualty statistics, on which national and regional road safety policy depends, has been repeatedly called into question. A technically feasible (although administratively challenging) solution is to pool data on road casualties from multiple sources, usually from both police and healthcare statistical agencies (Lyons *et al.*, 2008; Jeffrey *et al.*, 2009).

Descriptive epidemiology of injury

As indicated earlier, the incidence of injury in the population is a matter for speculation. In the UK, for example, although a fairly sophisticated system of routine national statistics exists, only the upper parts of the injury pyramid are reasonably well quantified.

A broad-brush description of injury epidemiology seeks to include information on the type of injury (whether unintentional or intentional), the severity (whether fatal or non-fatal) and the socio-economic patterns and the age groups affected (whether children or adults). Some estimate of financial cost is often added if this is available. These variables may be further refined depending on the availability of more detailed information.

Here is a thumbnail sketch of the epidemiology of injury in a typical (although unspecified) Western European country:

❑ Of all child injury deaths, around two-thirds are unintentional and one-third are intentional.

❏ Around two-thirds of unintentional deaths occur on the roads, the remainder occurring in the home or other settings.

❏ Non-fatal childhood injuries that result in hospital admissions greatly outnumber fatal injuries.

❏ Non-fatal childhood injuries that result in presentations to primary care or to EDs greatly outnumber hospitalisations due to injury.

This epidemiological summary is, of course, extremely crude. It fails to highlight five specific variables or risk factors that exert a striking influence on injury rates and are therefore important for prevention. These are geography, gender, socio-economic status, time and developmental stage (approximating to age).

Geography

International variations in injury mortality are striking and difficult to interpret due to doubts about the consistency of data validity between countries (see the discussion of the international dimension in Chapter 10). Even within countries, there are variations. While the overall pattern of injury is remarkably consistent geographically, there are some variations in injury epidemiology across the UK. Northern Ireland and Scotland (Figure 2.3) tend to suffer higher injury mortality rates than other parts of the UK, perhaps reflecting either a greater concentration of social deprivation in these areas or a higher prevalence of behavioural risk factors such as alcohol misuse (or both). The possibility of artefactual variation caused by differences in data collection, classification and reporting, as well as data quality, cannot be excluded.

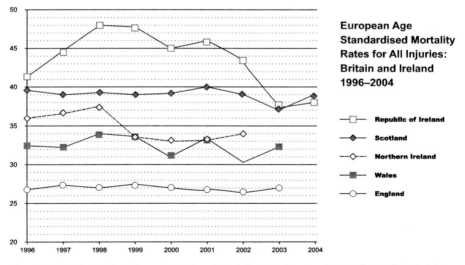

Figure 2.3 Variation in injury mortality rates between the countries of the British Isles. Reproduced by kind permission of the injury Observatory for Britain and Ireland. See: www.injuryobservatory.net/documents/Country_trends.xls (accessed 7 February 2011).

Other geographical influences on injury risk include urban–rural differences, which produce obvious and direct effects such as a greater number of agricultural injuries in the countryside, as well as indirect effects such as more serious road casualties resulting from the higher speeds that vehicles achieve on rural roads. Urban areas tend to contain more densely populated communities that experience severe social deprivation, and these risk factors are reflected in injury rates.

Gender

Numerous studies have reported that boys are at higher risk from most types of injury than girls. An exception may be house fire injuries, many of which occur at night when residents are asleep, and children of both genders are at equal risk. The gender difference in injury risk is non-existent in the neonate, increases with age and is already noticeable in infancy for some types of injury, including head injury. The phenomenon is so consistent and well recognised that many readers may assume, wrongly, that it is well researched and understood. In fact, the explanation is far from clear. Hypotheses abound, and these relate to physical and cognitive development, motor coordination, activity levels, a greater propensity for risk-taking or a greater exposure to hazardous environments (or some combination of these factors) in males. Injury-prone behaviour in boys may be reinforced by parental expectations and by media and advertising pressures. Oddly, the male excess in childhood risk of unintentional injury mortality in some age and causal categories appears to have been declining in recent years, again for reasons that are obscure (Pearson *et al.*, 2009). This changing pattern may have implications for prevention.

Socio-economic status

Injury is one of the most strongly socially patterned of all disorders of childhood. This is important for public health because whenever a disorder displays this epidemiological characteristic, it is likely to be due to (or at least mediated by) environmental factors, and is thus potentially preventable. Death rates from injury to children from the most deprived areas in Scotland, for example, are around three times those from more affluent areas (Figure 2.4). In other countries, variables such as race and education are essentially proxies for socio-economic status and show the same correlation with injury, although the strength of the association varies with injury type and severity. As with gender, the reason for this phenomenon is unclear and reflects a combination of environmental, behavioural and other risks interacting in complex ways. An association between deprivation and child injury mortality is a fairly consistent finding, although the degree of correlation varies between studies. Fire-related injuries are especially highly correlated with deprivation, presumably because they are so often caused by a toxic mix factors that are, in turn, closely associated with poverty such as poor housing, flammable furniture, smoking and alcohol.

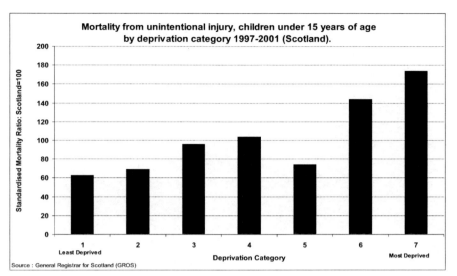

Figure 2.4 Correlation of child injury death with social deprivation in Scotland, 1997–2001.

By contrast, the socio-economic distribution of non-fatal injuries is much less clear-cut. Injuries to children presenting a hospital ED in Scotland, for example, did not seem to be so strongly socially patterned when the socio-economic character-istics of the population at risk were taken into account (Brown *et al.*, 2005).

The correlation between the incidence of child pedestrian casualties and social deprivation is especially noteworthy. White *et al.* (2000) found that the risk of death in Scotland was four times higher in children of the lowest socio-economic status than the highest, and that this mortality gap was widening over time. These findings were largely confirmed in an analysis of English data (Graham *et al.*, 2005). The authors observed that the deprivation effect on children was twice that on adults, and that these individual-level correlations were separate from a locality effect.

How does this increased pedestrian casualty risk to children from poorer back-grounds arise? Christie (1995) offered several plausible hypotheses:

❑ higher exposure rates due to more children from deprived areas being outside rather than inside vehicles;
❑ less adult supervision of children exposed to the traffic environment;
❑ lower educational levels and thus an inadequate understanding of road safety;
❑ increased susceptibility due to more risky behavioural patterns.

A combination of some or all of these factors may be at work. They are cited here because they could equally well apply to many other types of childhood injury.

Time

Although childhood injury mortality is expected to rise up the global league table in the coming decades, the picture varies greatly from country to country. Some of this reflects methodological weaknesses or random variation, but some is almost certainly real.

Injury mortality rates – especially in children – have been declining steadily in the UK and many other developed countries in recent decades. In some locations, the decline has been remarkable and unprecedented. In Scotland, for example, the proportional decline in road and home fatalities has been around 80% and 60%, respectively. These trends are usually interpreted as a major success for prevention. This has prompted some observers to suggest that injury is no longer a major public health challenge.

HEATED DEBATE No. 3:
Declining mortality from injury – victory at last?

Does the declining mortality from child injury in developed countries mean we should no longer take the problem seriously? After all, the public health agenda is a crowded one with many other pressing health problems vying for attention. Since we appear to have achieved considerable collective success in counteracting injuries, isn't it time to move on?

Opponents of that view are able to muster several counterarguments:

○ Although injury mortality rates have been declining in most developed countries, proportional mortality (relative to other causes of death) from injury has changed less, with the result that injury remains the largest single cause of mortality for adolescents and young adults in many parts of the world.

○ Even where injury mortality rates are declining rapidly, cause-specific injury mortality rates are not all falling consistently, with intentional injury mortality set to overtake unintentional mortality within a decade or two if current UK trends continue.

○ Mortality is only the tip of the injury iceberg. For every death, there are at least 10 hospitalisations (and, in some countries, at least 100) and many times that number of injuries treated as outpatients and in schools, workplaces and other settings. And these figures fail to capture the many injuries that cause lifelong disability and distress for individuals and their families.

○ Declining mortality could reflect declining case fatality rates due to better healthcare, especially acute trauma care in increasingly skilled regional clinical facilities. The assumption that declining injury mortality reflects declining incidence (about which we have little information) could be a false one.

○ Research evidence on the 'implementation gap' (what we could achieve minus what we have achieved) from the USA and elsewhere suggests that a further substantial proportion (30–50%) of injury deaths may be avoidable through the more consistent, vigorous and sustained application of existing knowledge.

○ The observed secular (long-term time) trends in injury death rates reinforce rather than undermine the idea that injuries are avoidable. In other words, prevention is more than merely a theoretical aspiration – the striking reduction in injury mortality over recent years in the developed world serves as an historical precedent for striving to avoid future injury deaths and acts as an inspirational spur for renewed preventive action.

○ As physical activity increases as a result of pro-exercise and anti-obesity policies, the risk of injury is likely to increase proportionately as we expose children more frequently to environmental hazards (on the roads, in parks, in playgrounds, in sport, etc). If that happens, the recent decline in injury mortality may well be reversed in the near future.

○ In global terms, injury mortality rates (particularly from road crashes) are still increasing and are predicted by the WHO to rise up the burden of disease league table in the coming decades (see Chapter 1). The international injury prevention community has a responsibility to disseminate knowledge of good practice to ensure that all parts of the world benefit from effective preventive strategies.

Conclusion
While the encouraging downward trend in child injury mortality is a welcome phenomenon that may, in part at least, represent successful preventive measures, continued downward pressure on incidence and severity remains a high priority for public health agencies and practitioners.

Age
Injury risk is developmentally determined, and age is a convenient, albeit fallible, proxy for development. With advancing age, children are exposed to changing injury risks for biological, behavioural, social and environmental reasons.

Infants ('babes-in-arms') are relatively well protected – although not by any means immune – from injury as a consequence of their being attached to or under the close observation of a parent (usually their mother) for most of the time. This conveniently contrived human microenvironment is essential for the care, nutrition, nurturing and general welfare of the dependent infant, but it soon gives way to a very different one after a year or so of life. Toddlers are naturally curious, and their mobility exposes them to a wide range of environmental hazards, mainly in the home. The transition to school is a key period when the child is at risk of injury on the road, in the school playground or during leisure activities such as swimming or cycling.

◼️LEARNING POINT

Injury risk is developmentally determined, and age is a convenient, albeit fallible, proxy for development. With advancing age, children are exposed to changing injury risks for biological, behavioural, social and environmental reasons.

Safety and child development
Children differ in their rate of development, but some degree of generalisation is permissible and helpful. The information shown in Table 2.1 is based on a guide

produced by the UK Royal Society for the Prevention of Accidents (RoSPA). It attempts to highlight some of the main child behavioural features associated with the various developmental stages up to age 8 years, along with some practical implications in the form of practitioner advice to parents or carers. More detailed advice of this kind is available from the Child Accident Prevention Trust (www.solihull.gov.uk/Attachments/Accidentsandchilddevelopment1.pdf accessed 7 February 2011).

Table 2.1 Injury prevention advice to parents/carers in relation to age.

Age	Development – what children do	Advice from practitioners
0–6 months	Wriggle and kick, grasp, suck, roll over.	Do not leave on a raised surface.
6 mths – 1 yr	Stand, sit, crawl, put things in mouth.	Keep small objects and dangerous substances out of reach.
1–2 years	Move about, reach things high up, and find hidden objects, walk, and climb.	Never leave alone, place hot drinks out of reach, use a fireguard and stair gates.
2–3 years	Be adventurous, climb higher, pull and twist things, watch and copy.	Place matches and lighters out of sight and reach. Be a good role model and be watchful.
3–4 years	Use grown-up things, be helpful, understand instructions, be adventurous, explore, walk downstairs alone.	Continue to be a good role model, keep being watchful but start safety training.
4–5 years	Play exciting games, can be independent, ride a bike, enjoy stories	They can actually plan to do things and carry it out. Rules are very important to them, as long as everybody keeps to the same ones. They enjoy learning. Continue safety training.
5–8 years	Will be subject to peer pressure and will still forget things.	Still need supervision, guidance and support.

Source: www.rospa.com/homesafety/adviceandinformation/childsafety/accidents-to-children.aspx (accessed 7 February 2011). Reproduced by kind permission of The Royal Society for the Prevention of Accidents (RoSPA).

As children become more mobile and mature, they become relentlessly curious about their environment and inevitably become exposed to hazards through their direct contact with inanimate objects (such as doors, walls and furniture), mechanical and electrical devices and the elements (particularly fire and water). All of this is enormously stimulating, enjoyable and educational for the developing and growing child. At the same time, the risk of injury, from the most trivial to the potentially fatal, is virtually ubiquitous. The result is that most toddlers are injured on a fairly regular basis, although most of the injuries are slight, cause transient pain or discomfort and are easily managed at home. Nevertheless, some injuries cause parental concern to the point where a decision is made to seek medical attention, and that usually involves a visit to the nearest ED.

Unsurprisingly, injury presentations to EDs (MacInnes and Stone, 2008) confirm that the maximal age of risk appears to be 1–3 years of age (Figure 2.5). Thereafter, the risk of injury is observed to decline throughout childhood until the adolescent years. These age-related patterns are remarkably consistent features of the epidemiology of injury across different populations, partly because they reflect the various stages of human development for which age is merely a rather crude if useful surrogate.

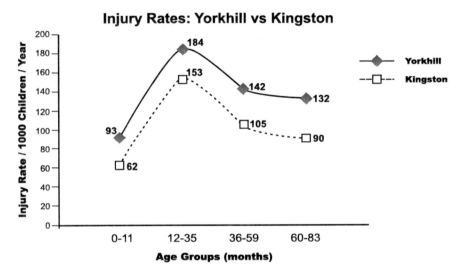

Figure 2.5 Trends in injury presentations to emergency departments at Yorkhill (Scotland) and Kingston (Canada) by age: rates per 1,000 population, calculated as an annual average over a 5-year period, 1997–2001. Canadian Hospitals Injury Reporting and Prevention Program data from west Glasgow postcode sectors only. Reprinted from Policies and Strategies to Promote Social Equity in Health. Stockholm: Institute of Future Studies by kind permission of BioMed Central. © 2008 MacInnes and Stone; licensee BioMed Central Ltd.

This developmental perspective on injury resonates with a broader trend within epidemiology that has implications for the whole of public health including all aspects of injury prevention. It has been dubbed the 'life cycle approach'.

A life cycle approach to injury epidemiology?

Epidemiologists have traditionally confined themselves to specific age groups or stages of the human life cycle. This can be both an advantage and an obstacle to progress. In recent times, the concept of life cycle epidemiology has been advocated (Ben-Shlomo and Kuh, 2002), a perspective that has proved highly productive in the injury field.

The anatomical location of injuries, for example, changes with circumstances and age. The case of falls illustrates this well. Young children often present with head injuries. Older children have greater awareness and psychomotor ability to protect themselves when falling and therefore present with more upper arm injuries. And in older adults, falls will often cause long bone injuries such as fracture of the neck of the femur.

Injury risk changes with age – or more precisely, developmental stage (see earlier). Children become increasingly active, mobile and interactive with the world around them as they grow, and that process is essential for normal development. That means that they will inevitably become exposed to a range of environmental hazards, initially in the home and later beyond its walls. Some of these hazards they will learn to cope with or avoid, others they will not, with consequences that range (in the majority) from mild, transient discomfort to more severe injury, disability or even death.

This dynamic and developmentally sensitive relationship between a child's age and the risk of injury (MacInnes and Stone, 2008) is reflected in the age distribution of injury incidence, as manifested in presentations to hospital EDs (Figure 2.5). It also has profound implications for policy-making and professional practice. A preventive programme aimed at the population of children as a whole is likely to fail unless an age-specific approach is adopted.

Injury types

Unintentional injuries form the bulk of all injuries in the population. These are usually subcategorised into transport, home, leisure and sport, work, and other injuries. The relative contribution of each of these depends on severity – road casualties contribute most to serious injuries, while home injuries more frequently result in non-fatal outcomes. The main injury types that children suffer include lacerations, contusions, sprains, fractures, burns and scalds, and ingestions.

In most countries, intentional injuries represent a minority of all injuries – although they may be gradually enlarging their contribution to the injury problem. Of these, suicide and deliberate self-harm are the most numerous forms, with interpersonal and group violence coming a long way behind in societies.

The relative proportions of injury types may change over time. In the UK and other European countries, fatal unintentional injuries in children have been declining for several decades, while intentional injuries have not; the result is that intentional injury mortality is becoming progressively more important epidemiologically. These time trends require careful monitoring as they may demand a changing public health response. Their existence must also be taken into account when the impact of countermeasures is being assessed.

The WHO (Peden et al., 2008) groups child injuries by five so-most called 'mechanisms': road traffic injuries (RTIs), drowning, burns, falls and poisoning. The definitions and epidemiological characteristics of these injuries are presented below in accordance with the WHO report.

Unintentional injury: epidemiology and natural history

Road traffic injuries (RTI)

Definition
Fatal or non-fatal injuries incurred as a result of a road traffic crash (RTC), i.e. a collision or incident that may or may not lead to injury, occurring on a public road and involving at least one moving vehicle.

Frequency and consequences
The scale of RTCs, and the misery they inflict, is startling. The Global Burden of Disease study estimated that nearly 1.3 million people were killed in RTCs in 2004 around the world and up to 50 million were injured or disabled. The highest rates were observed in the African and Eastern Mediterranean regions. About a fifth of the RTC deaths were in children. Although there have been downward trends in these figures in several developed countries, RTC injuries are predicted to rise in the next few years to be the fifth leading cause of death worldwide and the seventh leading cause of DALYs lost (Mathers and Loncar, 2005). The global economic impact is huge, amounting to an estimated US$518 billion per annum (Jacobs *et al.*, 2000).

RTIs make the largest single contribution to childhood injury mortality – over a quarter of a million deaths (about 30% of all injury fatalities and about 2% of all child deaths) in children and young people (0–19 years) were attributed to this cause in 2004. More than 90% occur in low- or middle-income countries. Although the data are incomplete, around a third of RTC deaths are pedestrians and the remainder are car occupants or users of two-wheeled vehicles. RTC mortality risk increases with age, peaking in the late teenage years, as does the male excess in mortality.

The prevalence of long-term consequences, including disability, from RTIs is hard to estimate but may be around 10 million (or 40 times the annual number of deaths), with pedestrian casualties having the poorest prognosis. Post-traumatic psychological syndromes are common in children following an RTI.

◀ LEARNING POINT ▬▬▬▬▬

RTIs make the largest single contribution to childhood injury mortality. More than 90% occur in low- or middle-income countries. Around a third of RTC deaths are pedestrians and the remainder are car occupants or users of two-wheeled vehicles.

Risk factors
Because children are growing, their tissues are more vulnerable to injury than those of adults, with smaller and younger children most liable to sustain damage. Their sensory facilities are still developing, and they are less aware of danger than adults. Cognitive immaturity results in poor decision-making and an inability to take effective evasive action. As children (especially boys) approach adolescence, impulsiveness

and risk-taking behaviour (as pedestrians, for example) may increase, either to exert a sense of control over their lives or to oppose authority. Peer pressure becomes an important influence on behaviour around this time. The male-to-female ratio of RTIs ranges from 3:1 to 5:1 for reasons that may relate to both exposure and behaviour (see earlier). As vehicle occupants, absent or inadequate restraints increase their risk of injury. Cycling children may be exposed to potentially lethal traffic, a risk that is heightened by not wearing helmets, lack of visibility and poor weather.

Lack of parental supervision of younger children is a risk factor, often related in turn to parental difficulties such as being a single or working parent or having physical or psychological disorders. Children from poorer backgrounds are at increased risk particularly of pedestrian injuries. Other risk factors include poor vehicle design, high traffic speeds and volumes, lack of off-road play areas, lack of safe public transport, and mixing of pedestrians, cyclists and heavy vehicles. Finally, the lack of high-quality and rapidly delivered pre-hospital and emergency trauma care, as well as of rehabilitation services, all contribute to high mortality and morbidity rates from RTIs.

Drowning

Definition

Drowning, whether fatal or non-fatal, is the process of experiencing respiratory impairment from submersion or immersion in a liquid.

Frequency and consequences

Nearly 400,000 people worldwide died in 2004 as a result of drowning, of whom almost half were under the age of 20 years. Children aged 1–4 years appear to be at highest risk. The drowning rate is six times higher in low- and middle-income than in high-income countries. The Western Pacific and African regions have the highest rates, with the Eastern Mediterranean region not far behind. Around 28% of all unintentional injury deaths in children are due to drowning. Like RTIs, drowning fatalities appear to have declined in high-income countries but not in the rest of the world. These figures may be substantial underestimates as data quality is poor and the Global Burden of Disease study excluded submersions as a result of floods and water transport incidents.

Non-fatal drownings are even harder to estimate but are thought to number 2–3 million per year. For each fatal incident, there may be four or more non-fatal drownings, and some of these, around 5%, result in serious long-term disabilities arising from respiratory or neurological deficits (Kemp and Sibert, 1991). The length of time submersed and the level of consciousness of the victim at the time of hospital admission seem to be a key predictor of prognosis. The psychosocial and economic consequences of drownings on families and communities may be lifelong.

Risk factors

Age is a risk factor for drowning, with very young children (apart from infants under 1 year who are usually unable to access water by themselves) and adolescents at highest risk. The male death rate is around double that of females, either due to greater exposure or to more risk-taking behaviour. Living in poverty or in rural areas seems to increase the risk, as does being a member of an ethnic minority. Some underlying medical disorders, such as epilepsy, autism and cardiac disease, increase the risk.

Lack of safety equipment, such as personal flotation devices, increases risk. Unsafe or overcrowded vessels, commonly seen in low-income countries, also place their passengers at risk. Alcohol consumption by parents or carers will impair supervision and increase risk.

The greatest risk of drowning arises from geography and consequent exposure to a body of water, both above and below ground. In poor countries, particularly those exposed to floods and tidal waves (such as with the Indian Ocean tsunami in 2004), most drownings occur during daily activities such as playing, working, going to school or washing. In affluent countries, most of the incidents occur in recreational settings such as unfenced swimming pools, lakes or rivers. Domestic baths are a serious hazard for young children if they are left unattended. Again, inadequate first aid and high-quality trauma care will reduce survival rates.

Burns

Definition

A burn is an injury to the skin or other organic tissue caused by thermal trauma from hot liquids (scalds), hot solids (contact burns), flames, radiation, radioactivity, electricity, friction or chemicals. Inhalation of hot or noxious gases may also cause inhalation burns or asphyxia, and may accompany skin burns. Skin burns may be superficial (first degree), partial thickness (second degree) or full thickness (third degree).

Frequency and consequences

Over 310,000 people died as a result of fire-related burns in 2004, of whom 30% were under the age of 20. The highest risk is in infants, and the death rates are highest in poorer countries, especially in Africa, South-East Asia and the Eastern Mediterranean. Fire-related deaths contribute the vast majority (above 90%) of all burn deaths, while most of the rest are due to scalds. The latter cause most of the morbidity due to burns. Smoke inhalation is the strongest determinant of mortality from house fires.

Disability, through scarring and contractures following such injuries, is relatively common. Other long-term sequelae include pain, anxiety, post-traumatic stress syndromes, phobias and social isolation (Esselman, 2007). Prognosis depends on several factors including the child's age, the body part affected, the proportion of the body surface area damaged, the timing and quality of healthcare provided and the extent of complications. Disfigurement of the face is especially problematic in terms of a child's self-esteem and social interaction. Younger children – while more vulnerable to tissue damage – appear more resilient over the long term than older age groups, with adolescents probably at highest risk of developing psychosocial disturbance following a severe burn. As with other injuries, the costs to individuals, the family, community and society as a whole can be enormous.

Risk factors

Age and developmental stage are key risk factors for burn injuries. Globally, infants are at highest risk of burn injuries, and the risk declines until the late teens, when it rises again. Very young children are both curious about their environment and lacking in the neuromotor skills to avoid harm. They tend to reach out and grasp hot objects, such as radiator pipes, have thin skin and poorly developed withdrawal reflexes, and are thus especially vulnerable to palm burns. Pre-school children experience scalds from hot liquids, mostly from cups of tea or coffee, that they pull down onto the upper parts of their body. Older children are more likely to be burned in serious fires outside the home.

Fatal burns, uniquely among injuries, are often more common in girls than in boys, while non-fatal burns are more evenly distributed between the genders. Girls tend to be more exposed to open fires and hot liquids in many parts of the world and may experience a higher risk still through the wearing of long, loose-fitting clothing in conservative societies. Other risk factors for burns include suffering from physical disability or poorly controlled epilepsy, being an asylum-seeker, living in a rural area and having parents who smoke. Poverty and its concomitants of low educational level, overcrowded living conditions, the use of unsafe cooking or heating equipment or fuel and inadequate supervision of children also contribute to increased risk.

▬(LEARNING POINT)─────────────────────────

In children, most of the mortality due to house fires is caused by smoke inhalation, while most of the morbidity is due to scalds caused by hot liquids.
● ●

Falls

Definition

A fall is an event that results in a person coming to rest inadvertently on the ground or floor or other lower level. By convention, some falls may be excluded from classification and reporting systems, such as those resulting from self-harm or assault, falls from animals or falls into water and machinery.

Frequency and consequences

Close to half a million people worldwide, mostly adults, died of falls in 2004. Non-fatal injury resulting from falls in children, by contrast, is the most common form of injury presentation to EDs. International comparisons are highly problematic because of classification and reporting differences. Low-income countries probably suffer much higher rates of falls, and more severe injuries, than high-income countries.

The severity of a fall is determined by three main factors – the anatomical site affected, the height of the fall, and the nature of the surface onto which the fall occurs. Falls from windows, balconies, roofs and trees are common, especially in older children. They are more likely to occur in the summer months when children are playing outdoors. Serious injuries, notably to the head, following falls from low heights should raise suspicion of possible abuse.

Falls are the leading cause of traumatic brain injury, whether fatal or non-fatal. Spinal cord, chest or abdominal injuries are rare and are usually associated with falls from considerable heights. Infants tend to suffer head injuries from falls, while older children injure their upper limbs as they attempt to protect themselves from the impact. Functional impairment or permanent disability, physical or psychological, may result form severe fall injuries. As with other forms of injury, the economic and other costs incurred following such injuries are substantial.

◾ LEARNING POINT ▬▬▬▬▬▬▬▬▬▬▬▬▬▬▬▬▬▬▬

The severity of a fall is determined by three main factors – the anatomical site affected, the height of the fall, and the nature of the surface onto which the fall occurs. Infants tend to suffer head injuries from falls, while older children injure their upper limbs as they attempt to protect themselves from the impact.

Risk factors

In a systematic review, Khambalia *et al.* (2006) identified age, gender and poverty as the most consistent independent risk factors for falls. Others included the height of the fall, the type of surface, the mechanism (whether dropped, falling down stairs, etc.) and the setting.

In infancy, falls are most likely to occur through being dropped or falling from furniture or car seats. In the pre-school age group, falls from steps or stairs, or from furniture or play equipment, become more common. In young children, there is a mismatch between their impulse to explore their surroundings and their capacity to assess and respond to danger. Later in childhood, falls from playground equipment of from being pushed are common, and risk-taking behaviour becomes increasingly prevalent.

There is a male excess in fall injury risk, due to patterns of exposure, behaviour and cultural expectations of gender-specific child behaviour by parents and carers.

Poverty seems to affect fall injury risk via overcrowding, hazards in the environment, single parenthood, unemployment, young maternal age, low maternal educational level, stress and other mental health problems of caregivers and inadequate access to healthcare. Certain consumer products are frequently involved in fall injuries. These include pushchairs, prams, baby walkers, high chairs, changing tables, cots, baby bouncers and bunk beds. Leisure products such as roller skates, roller shoes ('Heelys'), trampolines, swings and bicycles have been implicated. Playground equipment, such as high climbing frames and hard surfaces, may also be sources of fall injuries.

Poisoning

Definition

Poisoning is an injury that results from exposure, through inhalation, ingestion, injection or absorption, to an exogenous substance that causes cellular damage or death. Poisoning may be acute or chronic – the latter is generally excluded from the concept of injury.

Frequency and consequences

Around a third of a million people died in 2004 worldwide as a result of unintentional poisoning. Most of these were adults, although one survey of selected middle- and high-income countries ranked it as the fourth leading cause of unintentional injury death in the age group 1–14 years, after RTCs, fires and drowning (Taft *et al.*, 2002). Low-income countries, notably in Africa, appear to have the highest mortality rates.

The substances most frequently involved in developed countries are medicines, recreational drugs, household products and pesticides. In developing countries, fuels such as kerosene and paraffin tend to be most often implicated. About five million people each year suffer snake bites, and children are at greater risk than adults in terms of both incidence and severity. In the tropics, especially during the rainy and harvesting seasons, snake bites are a particular hazard, and the fatality rate can be as high as 25% in some countries. That is something of a special case: the vast majority of poisonings are non-fatal, and case fatality rates in hospitalised patients are usually low. The availability of prompt and effective treatment will clearly influence immediate prognosis. There are, however, few data on long-term prognosis or costs.

◄ LEARNING POINT ▶

The substances most frequently involved poisonings in developed countries are medicines, recreational drugs, household products and pesticides. In developing countries, fuels such as kerosene and paraffin tend to be most often implicated.

• •

Risk factors

As with other injuries, the triad of age, gender and poverty comprises the main epidemiological risk factors for poisonings. Infants, being closest to the ground, are at highest risk of ingesting toxins within easy reach, and they suffer the highest risk of death. By the age of 2 years, the risk of poisoning (although not of dying) has risen sharply as children are able to venture further afield. Poisoning rates seem to fall thereafter until adolescence, when the impact of alcohol, recreational drugs and self-harm appears on the horizon. Poisoning is generally more common in boys than in girls, at least in the younger age groups. Poverty is a consistent risk factor for poisoning around the world, first because of a greater exposure to hazardous substances in poorer homes, and second, because of related factors such as carers' low educational level and inadequate service provision.

The nature of the poisonous substance can play a role. Children are more likely to ingest liquid than solid medications, for example, as well as substances with an attractive, colourful appearance and a sweet taste. Inadequate or inappropriate storage of harmful substances in containers without child-resistant closures poses a greater risk. Countries that lack adequate regulations for the manufacture, packaging, distribution, storage and disposal of toxic substances place their children at higher risk of poisoning. Poison information or control centres are an invaluable resource but simply do not exist in many parts of the world.

Intentional injuries: epidemiology and natural history
Suicide

Most intentional injuries are self-inflicted rather than due to assault. Suicide, like injury as a whole, is a global public health problem and is by far the largest component of intentional injuries in most countries, except in early childhood, when suicide is rare. Unlike injury as a whole, the epidemiological trend of suicide, especially in young people, seems to have been upward – around 60% since 1950 (Guo and Harstall, 2004) – in most parts of the world, including developed countries. Moreover, suicide rates are generally higher in developed than in undeveloped countries, perhaps reflecting demographic or reporting differences. All of these figures are subject to controversy due to doubts surrounding data quality. Suicide remains a taboo subject in many cultures, and national statistics may be highly misleading. Underreporting and misclassification are common.

Males are at least four times more likely to die of suicide than females, although females are more likely to self-harm. Adolescents in their late teens are the highest risk age group in early life. Children under 15 years have about a tenth of the risk of suicide of their older peers, but the rates in younger groups appear to have been rising in recent decades, possibly due to more accurate reporting. Suicide means vary according to the country, culture and age – firearms, poisoning and strangling are most frequently used methods in the USA, for example, due to the widespread availability of guns in that country. There are several, perhaps hundreds, of suicide attempts (deliberate self-harm or parasuicide) for every one that succeeds. Suicidal thinking, often associated with depression (once erroneously believed to be extremely rare in childhood) is a common risk precursor. Suicide or self-harm may be more impulsive in children than in older people.

◄█LEARNING POINT►─────────────────────────

Adolescents in their late teens are the highest risk age group for suicide in young people. Males are at least four times more likely to die of suicide than females, although females are more likely to self-harm.

• •

Suicide is associated with a range of risk factors relating to physical, mental and social health, some of which operate in the very early years of life. A large retrospective study of middle-aged adults registering with the Kaiser Permanente healthcare plan in California has reported high frequencies of adverse childhood experiences (such as parental depression, suicide and family violence) in patients suffering from presenting with depression, suicidal thinking and substance misuse (Felitti *et al.*, 1998). Around 90% of suicide victims have a history of depression, other mental illness or substance abuse, and many have a history of previous suicide attempts.

Deliberate self-harm

The prevalence of deliberate self-harm is hard to determine but could be in the region of as high as 1 in 10 teenagers, particularly females (Hawton *et al.*, 2002). The Child and Adolescent Self-harm in Europe (CASE) study reported that over 70% of a large sample (30,000) of 15–16-year-olds admitted, via an anonymous questionnaire, to having self-harmed at some point in their lives 'to get relief from a terrible state of mind' (Madge *et al.*, 2008). Deliberate self-harm seems to be an emotional response to overwhelming stress related to low self-esteem or an event such as bereavement or intrafamily conflict, although it may, in some cases, be linked to a concurrent mental disorder such as depression. Cutting, for example, induces mood change through the release of endorphins. Girls who self-harm outnumber boys by 6.5 to 1 (Hawton and Harris, 2008). Children in care or custody appear to be at higher risk.

Interpersonal violence

Violence, like injury as a whole, is a public health challenge that causes death, injury, disability and suffering to large numbers of people. It places heavy demands on healthcare services and a large burden of cost on society. Yet it can be prevented.

Causes of violence

Violence takes many forms. Its definition and causes are subject to intense debate. Much public concern about violence focuses on adolescence, partly at least because that is the stage of the life cycle when the use of violence is liable to inflict the most severe injuries.

Tremblay (2006) has argued that violence is ubiquitous in human societies and that violence is thus a relative concept. He further asserts that violence has to be viewed in the context of developmental trajectories. Longitudinal data suggest that the onset of physical aggression occurs in childhood, probably before the age of 2 years, and steadily declines in most children. In other words, aggression is a developmentally appropriate behaviour in very young children. A small proportion (3–5%) maintain high levels of aggression into adolescence. Tremblay proposes that, while some degree of aggression is normal, children need to learn alternative problem-solving strategies. Efforts to 'correct' violent behaviour in later life are virtually doomed to failure.

In parallel with our enlarging understanding of the developmental origins of violence, it is becoming clear that the risk factors for both perpetrators and victims tend to overlap. That phenomenon reflects both the similar environmental and cultural milieu to which both parties have been exposed and the intergenerational nature of violent behaviour among young adults, whether directed towards peers or children.

Causes of violence against children

All researchers agree that the causes of violence are multiple and complex. The following (modified) list of factors that may contribute to the risk of assault and interpersonal violence was proposed by Rosenberg and Mercy (1991):

- ❑ biological (male sex, young age, brain disorder);
- ❑ psychological (previous abuse, violent behaviour by parents);
- ❑ cultural (male attitudes, media glorification);
- ❑ structural (poverty, racism);
- ❑ synergistic (substance misuse).

Hosking and Walsh (2005), in their literature review of violence research, proposed a striking metaphor of 'bombs with fuses' to describe violent offenders. They suggested that violence resulted from a combination of individual propensity – 'bombs' – with familial, community or societal factors – 'fuses'. The individual factors arise from negative early childhood experiences that interfere with normal development (neurophysiological as well as emotional) and the capacity to empathise with others. Empathy, they argue, is the greatest single inhibitor of the propensity to violence, and empathy fails to develop when parents or carers are unable to attune with their infants. Absence of attunement combined with harsh discipline is 'a recipe for violent, antisocial offspring'. The external trigger factors are numerous and include the stress of poverty, alcohol and drug misuse, and peer pressure.

Child maltreatment

Although children have been abused and killed, mainly by their parents, throughout human history, the statutory agencies seemed extraordinary reluctant to confront the problem until the second half of the 20th century when an American paediatrician

(Kempe *et al.*, 1962) coined the phrase 'the battered baby syndrome' and was met with widespread scepticism. In the UK, the death in 1973 of Maria Colwell at the hands of her stepfather ignited public opinion. Following that case, the government issued guidelines to local authorities on the management of 'non-accidental injury' in what turned out to be a largely futile attempt to avoid a repetition.

Child maltreatment is difficult to study and quantify due to its disturbing nature and consequent underreporting. It seems likely that at least half of child abuse and neglect deaths are not reported as such (Crume *et al.*, 2002). Children under the age of 3 years are at the highest risk of potentially fatal maltreatment. The vast majority of the perpetrators are the parents, more frequently fathers than mothers. Family stress, including poverty, substance misuse and a history of parents having been abused as children, are all risk factors.

◢LEARNING POINT

Child maltreatment is difficult to study due to its disturbing nature and consequent under-reporting. It seems likely that at least half of child abuse and neglect deaths are not reported as such. Children under the age of 3 are at the highest risk of potentially fatal maltreatment.

Prevalence estimates vary widely even within a country. Children with disabilities may be at higher risk. Furthermore, both attitudes and behaviour may be changing over time. In the UK, for example, a survey (Creighton and Russell, 1995) of the childhood experiences of a national sample of adults aged 18–45 reported that 35% said that they had been hit with an implement. Only 7% felt that it was acceptable to do that to a child at the time of the survey.

In a retrospective study (for the National Society for the Prevention of Cruelty to Children [NSPCC]) of around 3,000 young adults in the UK, Cawson *et al.* (2000) estimated that 16% (1 in 6) of children experienced 'serious maltreatment' by their parents at some time in their childhood. Of these, one third experienced more than one type of maltreatment. Serious maltreatment was defined as one or more of the following: physical violence, sexual abuse, absence of care or supervision, and emotional abuse. When moderate maltreatment was added to this, the prevalence rose to 38%. These are probably the most complete and detailed epidemiological data on the frequency of child abuse in the UK that are available.

Consequences of child maltreatment

Lazenbatt (2010) reviewed the research literature on the physical, mental and social consequences, along with their implications for practice and policy, of child abuse for the NSPCC. The most easily diagnosable clinical manifestations of abuse include bruising, lacerations, burns and scalds, fractures, subdural haemorrhage (due to skull injuries or being violently shaken), genital injuries and infections (including syphilis and HIV/AIDS). Subtler effects of abuse include growth faltering, developmental delay, headaches, obesity and endocrine disorders.

The longer term consequences of abuse are multiple and wide-ranging, depending on the frequency, severity and duration of the abuse as well as on the resilience of the child. Apart from the immediate, direct effects of injury and associated emotional disturbance, abuse impairs a child's physical and mental health and intellectual, emotional and social development. In later childhood, adolescence and young adulthood, it is associated with aggressive behaviour, poor educational outcomes, post-traumatic stress disorder (PTSD), depression, deliberate self-harm, suicide, violent criminal activity, poor relationships with peers, unemployment and homelessness. High-risk behaviours, including addictions to nicotine, drugs and alcohol, are common, with adverse consequences for health later in life. Moreover, the abuse is often transmitted to the next generation when the victims become parents who are less likely to provide good parenting and more likely to abuse their own children.

◖LEARNING POINT ◗
Apart from the immediate, direct effects of injury and associated emotional disturbance, abuse impairs a child's physical and mental health and intellectual, emotional and social development.

Group (collective) violence

Some readers may be surprised to find a section on group or collective violence, such as war and terrorism, in this book. After all, there seems little that the individual practitioner or policy-maker can do to prevent outbreaks of violence on such a large scale. This fatalism verging on nihilism is reminiscent of the widespread attitude to unintentional injury that held sway for so long. In reality, despite the scale of the challenge and the limited evidence base for prevention, countermeasures are available and these are all too rarely deployed.

A specifically public health perspective on mass violence and its prevention has recently begun to emerge. Collective violence has been defined (Dahlberg and Krug, 2002, p. 215) as:

> the instrumental use of violence by people who identify themselves as members of a group – whether this group is transitory or has a more permanent identity – against another group or set of individuals, in order to achieve political, economic or social objectives.

The WHO has identified three levels of group or mass violence:
- ❑ wars, terrorism or other violent political conflicts that occur between or within states;
- ❑ state-perpetrated violence such as genocide and torture;
- ❑ organised violent crime such as banditry and gang warfare.

This may be paraphrased as political violence, state-sponsored repressive violence, mass criminal violence. Of these, only warfare is regarded as having (potentially) a legal basis. The Geneva Convention of 1949 attempted to set out a code of military conduct that should be adhered to by all parties involved in armed conflict.

Probably the most extreme form of mass violence is genocide. This is defined by the 1948 Convention on the Prevention and Punishment of the Crime of Genocide (promulgated in the wake of the Nazi Holocaust) as 'Any ... acts committed with intent to destroy, in whole or in part, a national, ethnical, racial or religious group.'

Scale of the problem of group violence

Hundreds of thousands and sometimes more people die from group violence every year. Accurate data are difficult to obtain, first, because many countries (especially in the developing world) lack sophisticated routine data systems, and second, because of bias. Bias is a particular problem when violence is committed in a political context by organised groups or states because of their desire to manipulate public opinion. The WHO places great emphasis on the value of data reported by humanitarian organisations such as Amnesty International and Human Rights Watch, ignoring the inconvenient fact that these non-governmental organisations may also be subject to external and internal pressures that bias the information that they publish.

◄LEARNING POINT▶────────────────────────────

Accurate data on group violence are difficult to obtain, first, because many countries lack sophisticated routine data systems, and second, because of bias. Bias is a particular problem when violence is committed in a political context by organised groups or states because of their desire to manipulate public opinion.

Some aspects of the epidemiological data are, however, clear. Group violence continues to take a heavy toll of lives and suffering around the world; poorer countries suffer disproportionately from group violence; the number of victims is rising over time; civilians are increasingly caught up in military conflicts; and most modern conflicts occur within rather than between states.

The Carnegie Commission on Preventing Deadly Conflict (1997) has sought to identify the main risk factors for states (or their populations) that are liable to become caught up in violent conflict. These include:

- ❏ political factors:
  - ○ a lack of democratic processes;
  - ○ unequal access to power;
- ❏ economic factors:
  - ○ grossly unequal distribution of resources;
  - ○ unequal access to resources;
  - ○ control over key natural resources;
  - ○ control over drug production or trading;
- ❏ societal and community factors:
  - ○ inequality between groups;

- ○ the fuelling of group fanaticism along ethnic, national or religious lines;
- ○ the ready availability of small arms and other weapons;
- ❑ demographic factors:
  - ○ rapid demographic change.

To these may be added globalisation, social inequality and technological advances in weaponry. The Commission emphasises that many of these risk factors can be identified before overt collective violence takes place and countermeasures are initiated.

The health consequences of conflict on a population may be obvious, but some are more subtle. In the former category are fatalities, non-fatal injuries, non-injury diseases such as infections and disabilities, both physical and mental. In the latter may be counted depression, suicide, substance misuse and antisocial behaviour.

At a social level, health consequences are bound to flow from the large number of displaced peoples caused by conflicts and the negative socio-economic impact of conflict on nations, communities, families and individuals. Industrial and agricultural infrastructure may be seriously damaged and an intolerable burden placed on health, educational and other services.

HEATED DEBATE 4: What causes injury – behaviour or environment?

In studying the aetiology of injury, epidemiologists and other scientists have identified two broad groups of causal or risk factors that have consistently emerged as important. These relate, on the one hand, to human behaviour and its consequences for lifestyle and risk-taking and, on the other, to the environment, whether physical, social or economic. But which of these is the more important? Finding an answer is essential for deciding on the most productive approach to prevention.

Because many injuries can be attributed to risk-taking behaviour, such as running across a busy road, speeding or failing to wear a cycle helmet or a car seat belt, logic dictates that behavioural factors should be the main focus both of aetiological studies and of preventive measures. This would be an oversimplification for the following reasons:

Human behaviour is partly determined by environment. If pedestrians are physically separated from traffic by a high barrier, children are less likely to be able to run across that road.

- ○ Environment, in turn, is partly determined by behaviour. Parents of toddlers who are especially boisterous or hyperactive will generally reorganise furnishings and other potential hazards around the home in such a way as to minimise exposure.
- ○ Behaviour and environment may be closely correlated and therefore difficult to disentangle. So-called 'accident-prone' children may suffer repeated injuries because they are continuously exposed to a hazardous environment rather than because of an innate propensity to take risks.
- ○ Even where behavioural factors predominate in increasing injury risk, countermeasures aimed at environmental modification may prove more effective than those designed to change behaviour. Exhorting drivers to adhere to speed limits, for example, is usually less successful than implementing traffic-calming schemes such as road humps or chicanes.

Injuries in children and young people are often ascribed to risk-taking behaviour. The risk-taking may be direct, such as running recklessly onto a road without checking for traffic, or indirect, such as misusing drugs or alcohol. A subtler form of risk-taking is being 'safety averse' by refusing to use safety devices such as car seat belts or cycle helmets. This is an area that is difficult to investigate due to its complexity and methodological challenges. The limited research that has been done has proved contradictory and unilluminating. A systematic review of the subject by Thomas *et al.* (2007, p. 9) concluded that 'risk taking behaviour as an umbrella concept cannot be regarded as useful model to explain accidental injury among young people'.

Conclusion
Although behavioural factors may make an important contribution to the causation of injuries, environmental factors may be at least as important. Countermeasures that bring about environmental change are thus more likely to be effective in preventing injuries than those seeking to alter human behaviour.

Mental health and physical injury

The term 'injury' is usually defined in purely physical terms – the acute and harmful transfer of energy from the environment to human tissue. Although 'trauma' is sometimes used to denote psychological disturbance, in mainstream clinical settings it is usually synonymous with 'injury'. Psychological factors or states may, however, be important as (1) causes and (2) consequences of injury.

Mental health and the aetiology of injury
Mental health has a role in the aetiology at two levels. First, the 'normal' acute emotional stress that everyone experiences in daily life increases the risk of injury. An example is frustration with the slow speed of traffic leading to dangerous driving (e.g. overtaking on a blind corner). Second, specific (usually severe) psychological disorders can predispose to injury risk. One example is psychotic depression, the presence of which is an established risk factor for both intentional injury (suicide or deliberate self-harm) and unintentional injury (e.g. road crashes). A second is attention deficit hyperactivity disorder in children, a psychological disorder that inevitably exposes affected children to greater risk of injury in the home, on the roads, at school and at play.

There is also a third role – that of psychological factors as *indirect* causes and consequences of injury. Chronic depression, for example, may contribute to an elevated injury risk through the taking of substances (such as alcohol or narcotics) or medication. Abusive or neglectful parenting will adversely affect the mental health of children in complex ways throughout their lives. Apart from the psychological morbidity that may ensue, including a propensity to aggressive or self-destructive behaviour, some of these effects will impair educational achievement, employment prospects and prosperity, all of which will increase the risks of poverty and the associated higher levels of injury incidence and mortality.

LEARNING POINT

Abusive or neglectful parenting will adversely affect the mental health of children throughout their lives, including inducing a propensity to aggressive or self-destructive behaviour. It may also impair educational achievement, employment prospects and prosperity, all of which will increase the risks of poverty and the associated higher levels of injury incidence and mortality.
• •

Mental health and the sequelae of injury

The most obvious instance of the psychological sequelae is the subsequent development of a cluster of symptoms collectively known as post-traumatic stress disorder (PTSD). Other such consequences might include the causation or triggering of psychoneurotic states such as anxiety, obsessive-compulsive disorders and reactive depression. Equally, more 'normal' (in clinical terms) emotional responses to injury that fall short of PTSD or other diagnoses are loss of self-confidence and/or self-esteem, which have, in turn, potentially serious social or economic consequences including loss of a job (reinforcing any a priori emotional disorders), producing longer term negative effects on mental well-being and diminution of earning power. Some degree of emotional distress is common in children of all ages following an injury, particularly when caused by an RTC or a fall from a height. Parents, too, may be extremely upset and guilty following the injury. Many of these sequelae are either masked or unrecognised by carers, particularly when children are involved, and services are generally not organised in a manner that offers routine emotional support to victims (Heptinstall, 1996).

The mental health consequences of child maltreatment are often profound and long-lasting. These were described earlier in this chapter (see 'Child maltreatment').

Implications

Recognising the links between injury and mental health has two key benefits. First, it offers additional insights into the aetiology of injury that could prove useful in designing countermeasures. Second, it provides additional pointers to the damaging consequences of injury that, when addressed by healthcare and other professionals, will enhance the prospects for successful amelioration and rehabilitation of the victims and their families.

SUMMARY OF CHAPTER 2

Epidemiology and natural history of injury

- The public health importance of injury derives from its epidemiology. In most developed countries, injuries are the largest single cause of death in children and young people and a major cause of morbidity.

- Declining injury mortality may reflect diminishing exposure, improved trauma care or increased survival rather than declining incidence, although injury prevention measures may have contributed to this trend.

- Globally, about 10% of all deaths and five of the 25 leading causes of death (road casualties, self-inflicted trauma, violence, drownings and war) are due to injury. Injury-related injury mortality is expected to rise up the Global Burden of Disease league table from around five million deaths annually to over eight million by 2020.

- The injury pyramid is a powerful model: it provides a graphic description of the relative proportions of injuries that present as different outcomes; it illustrates the relatively small number of more serious outcomes in the context of the totality of injury; and it shows how the various components of the pyramid relate to each other in time.

- Injury mortality and hospitalisation rates contain numerous sources of error, including diagnostic inaccuracy, misclassification and bias. Nevertheless, these data are usually the most widely available indicators of injury occurrence that exist and are thus useful epidemiologically.

- Large numbers of injuries present to health services in ways that are not captured by routine statistics. Injuries to children may be self-treated or treated by parents or carers, or by community practitioners.

- Because injury is such a universal human experience, we need to distinguish between injury that is significant from a preventive perspective and injury that is not. Setting a threshold of severity above which we record injury is one way of achieving this.

- Most fatal injuries are unintentional. Of these, most occur on the roads, with the remainder occurring in homes, at play and in a variety of other settings. There are more injury-related hospitalisations than deaths. emergency department visits comprise the largest number of injury events resulting in contact with the healthcare services.

- While boys are generally at higher risk of injury than girls, the gender difference in injury risk is non-existent in neonates and increases with age. Although the phenomenon is consistent and well recognised, the explanation remains unclear.

- Injury is socially patterned. Death rates from injury to children from the most deprived areas are higher than those from more affluent areas.

- Injury risk is developmentally determined. Infants are relatively well protected from injury due to their being attached to or under the close observation of a parent. This human microenvironment soon gives way to a very different one after a year or so of life.

- Most intentional injuries are self-inflicted rather than due to assault. Suicide, like injury as a whole, is a global public health problem. Unlike injury as a whole, the epidemiological trend of suicide, especially in young people, seems to have been upward.

■ The prevalence of deliberate self-harm could be high as one in 10 young people aged 11–25. The Child and Adolescent Self-harm in Europe study reported that over 70% of a large sample of 15–16-year-olds admitted to having self-harmed at some point in their lives.

■ Violence is becoming recognised as a public health challenge that causes death, injury, disability and suffering to large numbers of people. It places heavy demands on healthcare services and imposes a large burden of cost on society. Yet it can be prevented.

■ Physical aggression starts in early childhood and declines in most children. In other words, aggression is a developmentally appropriate behaviour in young children, a small proportion of whom maintain high levels of aggression into adolescence.

■ Empathy is probably the greatest single inhibitor of the propensity to violence, and empathy fails to develop when parents or carers are unable to attune with their infants. Absence of attunement combined with harsh discipline is a recipe for violent, antisocial offspring.

■ Group violence continues to take a heavy toll of lives and suffering around the world; poorer countries suffer disproportionately from group violence; the number of victims is rising over time; civilians are increasingly caught up in military conflicts; and most modern conflicts occur within rather than between states.

■ Mental health has a role in the aetiology of most types of injury at two levels. First, the 'normal' acute emotional stress that everyone experiences in daily life increases the risk of injury. Second, specific (usually severe) psychological disorders can predispose to injury risk.

CHAPTER 3

Preventive approaches to injury

Learning objectives

- To have a basic understanding of the public health approach to injury
- To be able to describe the nature of injury surveillance, its uses, advantages and drawbacks, and key quality criteria
- To be aware of the various approaches, including theoretical frameworks, for preventing injuries
- To have an outline knowledge of the main components of injury prevention policy-making

The public health approach

It is often said that effective injury prevention demands a public health approach. What does this mean? At one level, it simply implies the adoption of a whole population perspective that depends on epidemiology as its underpinning science – although not at the expense of other disciplinary methods such as engineering, psychology and ergonomics. But the public health approach also implies the application of a particular type of systematic, evidence-based analysis of highly complex health problems.

Public health is the promotion of health and the prevention of disease (including injury) in the population through the organised efforts of society. The public health approach to any health challenge involves taking a considered, systematic series of steps – expressed below as questions – as follows:

- ❑ What is the problem (nature, scale, consequences, costs)?
- ❑ What are its key determinants (risk factors, causes)?
- ❑ What interventions are known to be effective in addressing it (evidence-based prevention or management)?
- ❑ What interventions are actually being implemented to address it (implementation)?
- ❑ How effectively and efficiently are these interventions being implemented (audit of measures of established efficacy or evaluation of measures of unknown efficacy)?

❏ What needs to be done to improve and monitor current implementation (recommendations for action)?

These six steps may be simplified to three: needs assessment ('diagnosis'), population-wide intervention ('treatment') and evaluation or monitoring ('follow-up'). These three steps represent the basic tasks of public health professionals and are analogous to the clinical approach to health problems that individual patients present to doctors and other healthcare practitioners:

❏ *Needs assessment* ('diagnosis'): What are the nature, scale, and determinants of the problem in the population?

❏ *Population-wide intervention* ('treatment'): What can and is being done to address it?

❏ *Evaluation or monitoring* ('follow-up'): How well are interventions currently being implemented, and how might they be improved?

■◖LEARNING POINT◗━━━━━━━━━━━━━━━━━━━━━━━━━

The three clinical tasks of clinical medicine – diagnosis, treatment and follow-up – may be scaled up to a population as the three tasks of public health – community diagnosis, population-wide intervention and evaluation or monitoring.
• •

Step 1: Needs assessment ('diagnosis')

This involves the analysis and interpretation of epidemiological data, whether these are obtained from routine statistical sources, injury surveillance systems or ad hoc surveys. This provides the public health practitioner with an indication of need or a '*community diagnosis*'. Getting this right is crucial as everything else will flow from it. The key elements of this process that will inform the community diagnosis are:

❏ clear specification and quantification of the problem or disorder under scrutiny (the numerator);

❏ accurate delineation of an appropriate population under study (the denominator);

❏ competent application of statistically and epidemiologically robust techniques for calculating and presenting rates or other data (analysis);

❏ Drawing valid conclusions about the problem and how it should be addressed (interpretation).

None of the above is straightforward, and details of how to set about such investigations may be found in standard epidemiological texts.

A specialised and extremely popular form of both needs assessment and monitoring in the injury prevention field is surveillance.

Injury surveillance, its uses, advantages and drawbacks, quality criteria

Surveillance (sometimes called monitoring) is a form of routine statistical analysis of injury data that has been shown to be helpful – some would say essential – in addressing the public health challenge of injury. At first sight, this may seem a similar activity to the analysis of routine statistics on death or health service presentations, and there is indeed some overlap, but there is also a subtle and crucial distinction.

Surveillance, as a public health tool, may be defined as the systematic, continuous and purposeful collection, analysis and reporting of data on a health topic with a view to the detection, reporting and, where appropriate, response to deviations from a predetermined norm. Crucially, this definition emphasises the link between data and intervention, implying that there is little point, in practical public health terms, in analysing the former as an end in itself (other than for research purposes).

Surveillance is therefore not merely passive data collection and analysis but is explicitly linked to action – either (or both) further investigation or the implementation of countermeasures. This idea of using data to trigger a response is familiar in the other fields of public health such as infectious disease control or environmental monitoring but remains relatively neglected in injury prevention.

◀ LEARNING POINT ▶

Surveillance is not merely passive data collection and analysis but is explicitly linked to action – either (or both) further investigation or the implementation of countermeasures.

The advantage of surveillance over other methods of statistical monitoring is that it ensures a degree of consistency over time and, sometimes, between locations where the surveillance system is in place. Clear inclusion and exclusion criteria can be specified, staff trained to apply them and a degree of quality control implemented. This consistency facilitates the identification of emerging trends, patterns or clusters that merit further investigation and perhaps preventive action. Once action has been taken, surveillance offers a means of evaluating or monitoring the impact, if any, on injury occurrence that has been achieved.

Surveillance seems a relatively simple concept but is in practice complex to deliver. The World Health Organization (WHO) has set out quality criteria for the implementation and evaluation of injury surveillance (Holder *et al.*, 2001), shown in Box 3.1.

What are the attributes of a good surveillance system?
Good surveillance systems have a number of attributes in common. These include the following.

Simplicity
The system should produce all the data needed but in a manner that is as simple and straightforward as possible. Forms and other records should be easily comprehensible and complete, and should not require staff to waste time unduly through the repeated entry of the same information. This is especially relevant when resources are limited and staff have other demands on their time.

> **BOX 3.1: World Health Organization quality criteria for injury surveillance**
> ✔ **Simplicity**
> ✔ **Flexibility**
> ✔ **Acceptability**
> ✔ **Reliability**
> ✔ **Utility**
> ✔ **Sustainability**
> ✔ **Timeliness**
> ✔ **Security and confidentiality**

Flexibility

The system should be amenable to change, especially when ongoing evaluation shows that change is necessary or desirable. For example, it should be possible to add information on another type of event to the surveillance system, or to change the target population so that a novel type of injury is captured.

Acceptability

The system will cease to work if people feel uncomfortable participating in it. Involving staff at each stage in the design, evaluation and improvement of data entry forms should help to ensure that they find them easy to complete and that they understand their purpose. It is also important to take account of the views and suggestions of end-users.

Reliability

End-users of data produced by a surveillance system should have complete confidence in the accuracy of the data. The system should therefore:

- ❑ fully record injury events (or cases), with all relevant information being included;
- ❑ classify injuries in accordance with accepted and explicit definitions;
- ❑ exclude non-injury events (e.g. chronic low back pain from osteoarthritis);
- ❑ detect all injury events within the relevant population (by ensuring that all the relevant hospitals or clinics are included) or be able to detect a representative sample of injury events that reflects the distribution of events in the whole population. (Sampling need not rely on *complete coverage*, but coverage must ensure that all types of injury event in all kinds of circumstances are equally covered.)

Utility

The system should be practical, efficient and affordable. It should not appear to place an unnecessary burden on an organisation's staff and budget.

Sustainability

The system should function with the minimum of effort and be easy to maintain and update, so that it will continue to serve its purpose long after it has been established.

Timeliness

The system should be able to generate up-to-date relevant information whenever that information is needed by the end-users.

Security and confidentiality

These are two further key features of a surveillance system. Records of individual cases should be kept entirely confidential. Surveillance reports should never reveal personal information on individuals. Moreover, the system should never expose personal information that could potentially embarrass the participants.

HEATED DEBATE No 5:
Is injury surveillance in emergency departments necessary?

The benefits of injury surveillance, like other forms of public health activity, cannot be taken for granted. After all, these systems are expensive and time-consuming. In an era of evidence-based public health, can their use in emergency departments (EDs) be justified on the basis of their documented impact?

Formal evaluations of injury surveillance systems are rare and, when they are conducted, highlight several deficiencies that have usually not been anticipated. There have been few published scientific studies on which to judge the impact of injury surveillance on either the process or the outcome of injury prevention (Stone *et al.*, 1998; Lyons *et al.*, 2002). The main drawback of surveillance is that it tends to be labour-intensive, even in an era of mass information technology, and that incurs a substantial cost. Unless the investment produces demonstrable returns in the form of either useful output for local planning or (ideally) reduced injury rates and/or severity over a reasonably short time-scale, the exercise may turn out to be unsustainable.

An evaluation of an injury surveillance system in a Scottish hospital concluded that too much attention had been paid to data collection at the expense of analysis and utilisation. The authors argued that surveillance is undermined if it is perceived by staff to be a research rather than a preventive tool. ED staff are not opposed to research – on the contrary, they depend on it for the effective discharge of their duties – but they simply have other, more immediate clinical priorities. To avoid this pitfall, they suggest that careful planning is required to ensure that three critical elements are in place – clinical supervision, data management, and intelligent analysis linked to intervention (Shipton and Stone, 2008).

Surveillance data derived from EDs are inevitably flawed. They are rarely population-based and usually contain inherent biases due to the unrepresentative nature of attenders in terms of age, gender, ethnicity, socio-economic position, time of day and place of residence (Stone *et al.*, 1999). Moreover, these data tend to describe injuries that are relatively minor and heal rapidly with few long-term sequelae. By contrast, deaths and hospitalisations are more distressing and expensive to society.

At the centre of the debate around ED-based surveillance lies a quasi-philosophical dispute. Advocates of surveillance claim that 'diagnosis should always precede treatment' and that surveillance in EDs offers us that crucial diagnostic tool on which preventive initiatives can be based. Opponents reject that view, pointing out that some clinical treatments are undertaken in the absence of a definitive diagnosis and that injury prevention can and should be implemented without the need for a detailed 'community diagnosis' that includes ED data.

Conclusion
Injury surveillance, in the widest sense, is an essential part of the public health process of 'community diagnosis'. ED-based surveillance has a role, but its benefits may have been exaggerated. The absence of ED-based surveillance should not be used as a fig leaf for preventive inactivity.

Step 2: Population-wide intervention ('treatment')
The second step in the public health approach requires a distillation of the research evidence to *identify efficacious interventions*, combined with a review of what is actually being done in practice. This evidence is generated by academic departments, research institutes and specialist centres through the performance of experiments of various types. Because the quality of published research studies is so variable, a particular form of research evaluation known as *critical appraisal* has been developed for this purpose. Critical appraisal of the scientific literature is the lynchpin of evidence-based practice (see Chapter 5).

Once the evidence base has been evaluated in this way and practical measures selected for implementation, the next step is to plan and create appropriately funded and supported mechanisms for delivery of those measures to the target population. This crucial stage is often neglected in public health, with the result that good intentions are never realised because recommendations, however meticulously crafted, are not properly implemented.

Step 3: Evaluation or monitoring ('follow-up')
The third public health step demands an evaluation, audit or monitoring mechanism to determine the strengths and weaknesses of current interventions with a view to making recommendations for the future. This is probably the least well understood and hence most neglected aspect of public health.

Evaluation, audit and monitoring are conceptually related terms. Evaluation simply means 'to determine the value of', although it is commonly used to describe a research method that compares a process or outcome with a predetermined objective or with a control group. Audit is used to assess the extent to which an intervention meets a standard that is regarded as good practice. Monitoring is loosely synonymous with surveillance (see 'Step 1: Needs assessment (diagnosis)', above), although the former term implies a more passive process of data collection and analysis than the latter.

The topic of evaluation is of such paramount importance, and so potentially contentious, that we will return to it at several points throughout this book.

Preventing injuries: theoretical frameworks

Contrary to a still-prevalent popular view, injuries are not random events. They are predictable and avoidable, perhaps to a greater extent than most other causes of mortality and morbidity in childhood. Over the past few decades, a large amount of research evidence has accumulated that is available to guide practitioners and policy-makers. Although more research is always required, the full implementation of the existing body of evidence could substantially reduce the incidence and impact of injury. Several studies from various countries have explored the issue of preventability and have concluded that at least a third of all childhood injury deaths could be avoided were interventions of known efficacy implemented (see Chapter 11). Assessing the extent of this implementation gap is difficult and controversial. Nevertheless, it seems reasonable to assume that a substantial further reduction in the incidence of injuries to children might be achievable in most countries. That would require the adoption of a systematic, strategic approach to injury prevention as a whole, starting with a robust conceptual foundation.

▄LEARNING POINT

Several studies have concluded that at least a third of all childhood injury deaths could be avoided were interventions of known efficacy fully implemented.

The public health literature conceptualises injury prevention in various ways. Two of the most popular are the three levels of prevention and the three Es.

Primary, secondary and tertiary prevention

Applying the classical model of preventive medicine, injury prevention may be primary, secondary or tertiary. These three levels are defined in relation to the stage of the natural history (course) of the condition.

Primary prevention is directed at the *pre-pathogenesis* phase of a disease – that is, before tissue damage has occurred. It involves the removal of circumstances, risks and hazards that lead to injury. Examples are child-resistant packaging, the manufacture of fire-resistant nightwear, the fitting of thermostatic mixing valves, and intensive parenting interventions.

Secondary prevention focuses on minimising the extent of tissue damage by intervening early in *pathogenesis*. It involves the reduction of injury severity in incidents that do happen. Examples are the fitting of seat belts, the wearing of motorcycle or bicycle helmets and the use of impact-absorbing playground surfaces.

Tertiary prevention seeks to alter the *post-pathogenesis* or recovery phase by mitigating the impact of tissue damage rather than preventing it. It involves providing the optimal treatment and rehabilitation of the injured person to minimise the consequences of injury. Examples are the administration of effective first aid, the rapid evacuation of injured patients to specialist care facilities, acute surgery and intensive care for trauma victims and the provision of services for the disabled injury victims.

The three (or four) Es

An alternative and widely quoted conceptualisation of injury prevention is the so-called three Es. These are (listed in reverse order of efficacy) education, enforcement of legislation and engineering (sometimes called environmental) measures.

◄ LEARNING POINT ──────────────────────────

A popular conceptualisation of injury prevention is the so-called three Es. These are (in reverse order of efficacy) education, enforcement of legislation and engineering (or environmental) measures.
• •

Education

Unless people are educated about safety, it is unreasonable to expect them to avoid injury through intuition or guesswork. And because so many injuries appear to result from risky behaviour, a rational response is to try to change that behaviour through either information dissemination or skill enhancement. Education may be directed at various groups – children, parents or carers, professionals and politicians – and may involve a range of methods to raise awareness, including media and advertising campaigns.

Enforcement

The term 'legislation' need not be restricted to laws passed by legislatures. It can also embrace product and service standards, industry codes of practice, local bylaws, purchasing protocols – and arguably even school rules. However defined, legislation that is not enforced, for whatever reason, is virtually pointless (apart from conveying collective social disapproval of a particular behaviour or activity). Enforcement, however, is labour-intensive and requires sustained commitment on the part of the statutory agencies such as the police and trading standards officers. That may, in turn, involve the redeployment of scarce resources in a manner that undermines competing responsibilities or antagonises colleagues, government or the public.

Engineering/environment

Advances in technology, building (including home design), road design, consumer product safety and other forms of engineering, in the broadest sense, all play a role in preventing injury. The wider environment – physical, social, emotional – is crucial to the generation or avoidance of injury risk. An important environmental dimension is poverty: the gradient of risk across children of different social classes is steeper for injury mortality than for many other causes of death in childhood, a phenomenon that may reflect the more hazardous environment of poorer localities. The three Es – education, enforcement and engineering – are sometimes supplemented by some more Es, including *empowerment* (of individuals, families and communities) and *evaluation* (to determine whether the action has been effective).

This last E is often overlooked, not merely for the reasons outlined earlier, but because it has a habit of revealing inconvenient truths. Among these may be counted the overwhelming evidence that educational campaigns and programmes tend to produce disappointing outcomes because they rely on active behavioural change. Passive engineering or environmental measures are usually much more efficacious, while legal enforcement lies somewhere between the two. That is problematic for policy-makers because educational measures are usually easier and more politically popular to implement than the other two strategies. There may be a compromise position, however, as educational campaigns can prepare public opinion – and therefore influence policy – for legislative or environmental change that would otherwise meet stiff resistance (Towner and Ward, 1998).

Conceptual models for facilitating injury prevention or control

Injury prevention, like other branches of public health, has flirted with several appealing theoretical frameworks over the years in an attempt to cope with the complexity of the challenge.

An example of an all-embracing model that offered a potentially useful way of thinking about public health in general and injury in particular injury was the Lalonde health field concept. Lalonde (1974), a Canadian Minister of Health, proposed four types of health determinants or fields: biology, lifestyle, environment and health services. This model proved especially helpful in focusing the minds of public health policy-makers on factors other than human behaviour. A renewed emphasis on both environment and healthcare injected novel thinking into strategy-making that had become bogged down in a rather narrow field of health promotion with its perceived dependency, at that time, on educating people to change their behaviour in health-promoting directions as the main means of pursuing the public health agenda.

> **Box 3.2: Lalonde's health field concept**
> ✔ **Environment** – all influences on health outside the human body and over which the individual has little or no control. This includes the physical and social environment
> ✔ **Human biology** – all aspects of health, physical and mental, developed within the human body as a result of organic make-up
> ✔ **Lifestyle** – the aggregation of personal decisions, over which the individual has control. Self-imposed risks created by unhealthy lifestyle choices can be said to contribute to, or cause, illness or death
> ✔ **Health care organisation** – the quantity, quality, arrangement, nature and relationships of people and resources in the provision of healthcare

Lalonde's report expressed complex ideas in a succinct and intuitively rational manner. For probably the first time, a government ministry had explicitly acknowledged the multifactorial nature of health and disease and committed itself to addressing the challenge in a comprehensive manner.

Public health experts and agencies found the model an exceptionally powerful tool for advocating a comprehensive approach to addressing contemporary health challenges. From a practical perspective, however, they soon discovered that their health improvement plans strained the Lalonde model close to breaking point. That led other writers to develop and embellish the concept in various ways in an attempt to introduce a greater degree of both complexity and specificity into the original.

The ultimate expression of this development was the more elaborate Evans and Stoddart (1990) formulation (Figure 3.1), which sought to identify the links between the various factors influencing health outcomes. Their insights could be summed up by the phrase 'everything matters'. That statement may be more or less factually correct but is arguably counterproductive owing to the sheer complexity of the numerous relationships between a startling array of variables.

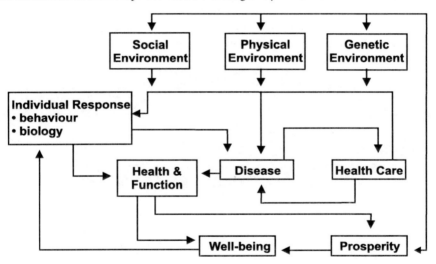

Figure 3.1 The Evans and Stoddart socio-ecological model of health promotion. Reprinted from Social Science and Medicine, 31, Robert G. Evans & Gregory L. Stoddart, Producing health, consuming health care, 1347–1363, 1990, with permission from Elsevier.

Dahlgren and Whitehead (1991) proposed a 'rainbow' that encompasses the wider social determinants of health along with those operating at the community, family and individual level (Figure 3.2). This proved to be a more intellectually coherent and has been highly influential in health promotion circle. To date, its application to injury prevention has been limited.

A variant of the 'rainbow' is the social ecological model (Figure 3.3) proposed by Dahlberg and Krug (2002). It has been highly influential in the evolving thinking around the prevention of injury and (particularly) violence of both the US Centers for Disease Control and the WHO.

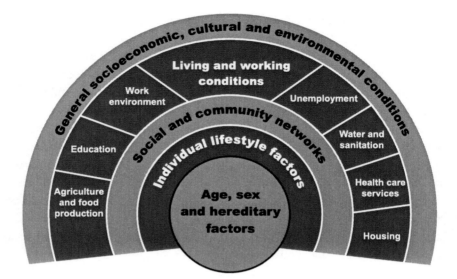

Figure 3.2 The Dahlgren and Whitehead model of health determinants. Reproduced by kind permission of the Institute for Future Studies, Stockholm.

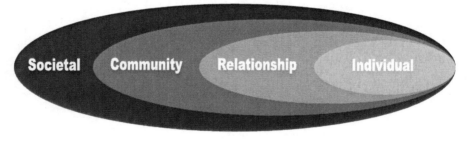

Figure 3.3 Dahlberg and Krug's social ecological model. Available from: www.who.int/violence_injury_prevention/violence/4th_milestones_meeting/publications/en/index.html (accessed 7 February 2011). Reproduced by kind permission of the WHO

This model represents the complex interplay between individual, relationship, community and societal factors that put people at risk. Prevention strategies should include developmentally appropriate activities that address multiple levels of the model across the lifespan.

The first level – *individual* – focuses on biological and personal factors that increase the risk of becoming either an injury victim or a perpetrator of violence. Examples include age, education, income, personality, illness and history of substance abuse.

The second level – *relationship* – includes factors that increase risk through human relationships of all kinds – with parents, siblings, peers, intimate partners and others. These relationships influence behaviour and contribute to exposure to risk.

The third level – *community* – encompasses the various settings (e.g. schools, workplaces and neighbourhoods) in which relationships occur and attempts to identify the characteristics of these settings that influence injury risk.

The fourth level – *societal* – addresses the broad societal factors that provide a context within which injury is more or less likely to occur. These factors include social and cultural norms, government policies and macroeconomic processes that influence social inequalities in the population.

Haddon Matrix

The name most closely associated with a systematic, public health approach to road safety is that of William Haddon, a physician and engineer (see Chapter 1). His eponymous matrix is an elegant and deceptively simple model for analysing and learning preventive lessons from road traffic crashes.

Haddon developed an earlier inspired idea of Gordon to apply the principles of infectious disease epidemiology to the superficially very different arena of road casualties. Gordon had suggested that the classic epidemiological triad of host, agent and environment could be applied to injuries. Haddon (1999) adapted and extended this notion (Figure 3.4) in a way that made sense to traffic engineers and public health professionals. The host was the injured person, the agent was the vehicle, and the environment was the context within which the crash took place. Both Gordon and Haddon recognised that injuries and infections were not as remote from each other as they might seem and that lessons learned form the prevention of the former could be applied successfully to the latter. Unlikely as it seemed, the experiment worked. The transition was seamless and effective.

Example of Pedestrian Head Injury			
•	Host	Agent	Environment
Pre-injury	Child running	Car speeding	Rain
Injury	Skull fracture	Bumper impact	Microbes
Post-injury	Coma	Unskilled first aid	Hospital care

Figure 3.4 The Haddon Matrix.

The Haddon Matrix contains nine cells created by the juxtaposition of three columns and three rows. When populated, these cells contain a rich seam of information on the sequence of events preceding and subsequent to the crash. This information may then be used to develop, in retrospect, preventive recommendations that might have prevented the crash, or at least the resulting injury or its consequences. An elaboration of the Haddon Matrix, proposed by

Runyan (1998), offered a means of adding further dimensions – including socio-economic ones – to the triad, although, arguably, these could be subsumed under the environment heading without tampering with the matrix itself.

The DPSEEA model

The DPSEEA model, by contrast, has a very different origin. Its roots lie in environmental health, a branch of public health that had traditionally been preoccupied with protection of the public from specific hazards in the air, water or food chain. DPSEEA is an acronym for drivers, pressures, states, exposures, effects and actions. These headings are interrelated in the form of sequential 'chains' or 'maps' that enable highly complex processes to be documented and analysed. The model was developed, with the endorsement of the WHO and the Children's Environmental Health Action Plan for Europe (CEHAPE) initiative, to encourage a new and much more joined-up, strategic approach to environment and health.

A variant, known as the modified DPSEEA model (Morris *et al.*, 2006), has been designed to offer practical solutions to real problems (Figure 3.5). It was created to embrace the local dimension of environmental health challenges and to recognise the socio-economic, behavioural and other influences that bear on the relationship between environment and health. The modification of the original model takes account of the socio-economic status of the population and other contextual factors.

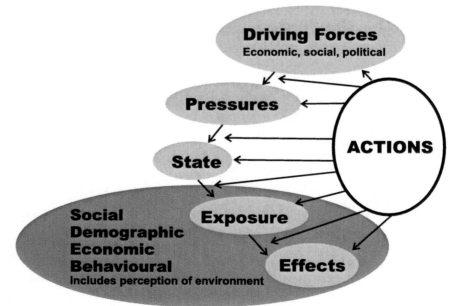

Figure 3.5 Modified DPSEEA model. Reprinted from Public Health, 120, Morris GP, Beck SA, Hanlon P, Robertson R (2006). Getting strategic about the environment and health, 2006, with permission from Elsevier.

Unlike the Haddon Matrix, the DPSEEA model explicitly considers 'actions', giving the approach clear policy relevance and practicality. The model can frame the problem, either quantitatively, qualitatively or both, in ways that highlight gaps and point to solutions.

Injury prevention policy-making

A curious paradox lies at the heart of injury prevention. On the one hand, the mainstream public health community has been slow to adopt it as a legitimate core concern or activity. The allocation of research funding to the field has lagged woefully behind that of other areas (Nicholl, 2006). On the other hand, injury prevention is one of the great historical success stories of public health, as vividly recounted by Hemenway (2009). Countless lives have been saved over many decades as a result of policies and practices that have greatly enhanced the safety of a wide range of activities. Much of this extremely effective work has been undertaken by engineers, architects, town planners and local officials out of the limelight and virtually unnoticed. Examples include the growing use of seat belts, drink-driving laws, child-resistant medicine containers, the wearing of helmets by motorcyclists, the implementation of building regulations, the application of product safety standards to children's clothing, nightwear and toys, the fitting of smoke detectors and sprinklers and the provision of parenting support programmes.

So it seems that injury prevention has been both scandalously neglected and hugely successful at the same time. How can we resolve this apparent contradiction? The answer is this: although injury prevention efforts have produced truly remarkable results on a breath-taking scale, many more lives could have been saved or improved either by the application of existing knowledge or by more focused and productive research. Moreover, that 'implementation gap' between knowledge and its application will remain a formidable challenge for public health in the future.

▪◖LEARNING POINT ◗━━━━━━━━━━━━━━━━━━━━━━

A paradox lies at the heart of injury prevention. On the one hand, the mainstream public health community has been slow to adopt it as a core activity. On the other hand, injury prevention is one of the great historical success stories of public health. Countless lives have been saved over many decades as a result of policies and practices that have greatly enhanced safety.

Role of politics, leadership and accountability

Rudolf Virchow, a German pathologist and one of the earliest 19th-century advocates of public health, asserted that 'politics is nothing else but medicine on a large scale', and nowhere is this truer than in the field of injury prevention. Politicians, despite the best of intentions, find themselves facing peculiar dilemmas in confronting injuries.

First, injuries may be politically invisible, because of the popular perception that 'accidents will happen'. Injuries may also be epidemiologically invisible due to the fragmented reporting of their various causes into road casualties, occupational injuries, suicides and others – a trap into which Sir Derek Wanless (Wanless, 2004) inadvertently fell when asked to consider the future of public health by the UK Treasury (see Chapter 11). Second, the notion of 'safety' is usually viewed through a criminal justice lens to the detriment of a public health approach. Third, the diversity and complexity of injuries ensures that they are the responsibility of multiple government departments and renders them immune to a single, clear and self-contained policy response. Finally, many injury prevention measures are somewhat counterintuitive in that they depend on environmental or legislative changes that appear to marginalise individual choice or, worse, have connotations of the 'nanny state' (see Chapter 12).

Overcoming these objections demands political leadership of a high order, the allocation of scarce public resources to the modification of infrastructure such as roads and playgrounds, and the adoption of a long-term perspective that extends well beyond the conventional electoral cycle of a few years.

Economic aspects

The huge cost of injuries to society is indisputable. Direct healthcare costs are probably about a tenth of global social costs. UK figures in 2002 were costs to the UK National Health Service of approximately £2 billion per year (of which £400 million relate to children), and global societal costs of at least £20 billion per year. Potentially, therefore, *prevention should represent an outstanding investment*.

One indirect measure of the cost savings of injury prevention is the UK Department of Transport's estimate of the costs incurred in a road fatality. Using their 'Willingness To Pay' method, the cost of a single life lost – or the value of prevention per casualty – is around £1.6 million (www.dft.gov.uk/pgr/statistics/datatablespublications/accidents/ accessed 7 February 2011). Unfortunately, the extent to which preventive measures generate long-term savings is uncertain as data are sparse as few cost–benefit analyses have been performed. Miller, using American data (Miller and Hendrie, 2005), estimated that $7 is saved for every $1 invested in prevention (Box 3.3). The returns in the UK and elsewhere may, however, be more modest as US healthcare costs are the highest in the world.

> **Box 3.3: Financial costs and benefits of selected child safety measures**
> ✓ **Every $45 child safety seat generates $1800 in benefits**
> ✓ **Every $30 booster seat generates $2000 in benefits**
> ✓ **Every $10 bicycle helmet generates $530 in benefits**
> ✓ **Every $30 smoke alarm generates $870 in benefits**
> ✓ **Paediatric injury prevention counselling at $9 per child generates $79 in benefits**

━◖LEARNING POINT━━━━━━━━━━━━━━━━━━━━━━━━━━━

American research estimates that $7 is saved for every $1 invested in prevention. Because of very high US healthcare costs, the equivalent figures elsewhere may, however, be more modest.
• •

The UK National Institute for Health and Clinical Excellence (NICE) commissioned a systematic review (Anderson and Moxham, 2009) of economic evaluations of legislation, regulation and standards in relation to a range of interventions. Only four survived intensive critical scrutiny: the compulsory wearing of bicycle helmets, the mandatory installation of domestic hot water thermostatic mixing valves, the mandatory installation of smoke detectors in homes, and the use of cameras to enforce speed limits. They concluded, with reservations about data quality, that all four were likely to be cost-effective.

HEATED DEBATE No 6: Targeted or universal prevention?

Epidemiological research has generated new insights into the way risk is distributed in the population. It is unarguable that different sectors of the population appear to experience different levels of risk. This has led public health professionals to seek ways of controlling specific risk factors with a view to prevention. A good example is coronary heart disease: millions of people identified as being at 'high risk' are taking medications to reduce serum cholesterol or blood pressure, with some fairly convincing evidence of benefit.

In the case of childhood injury, we know that males, the disadvantaged and children of single parents, especially young mothers, are more likely to suffer certain types of injury, and that injury severity is also sometimes linked to some risk factors. Moreover, parenting support programmes, such as the Nurse–Family Partnership, that are targeted at these high-risk groups appear to have a positive impact in promoting parenting skills and producing healthier outcomes, including lower injury rates (Kendrick *et al.*, 2007). The temptation for public health agencies is therefore to build on this research by targeting interventions at high-risk groups. This is logical, appealing – and misguided. The pros and cons of targeting, as a public health strategy, may be summarised as follows.

The case for targeting

Targeting high-risk groups is often advocated as a public health strategy on the following grounds:

○ Available resources are always limited (especially in the UK in 2010–14), and it is therefore better to target interventions at those most in need as they are clearly deserving of greater help. This is essentially a moral and political rather than a scientific or economic argument.

○ Targeting interventions at those at highest risk appears rational and logical. Outcomes are assumed to be better in high-risk groups as these appear offer more scope for improved outcomes (although the potential for a spurious improvement through regression to the mean is often overlooked).

○ The research evidence base (randomised controlled trials) appears to support targeted interventions, while a universal approach risks diluting any impact. That is because researchers strive to define population subgroups in which they can test hypotheses. The result is that universal approaches have been underresearched.

○ More educated and affluent individuals, families and groups are believed to be more likely than disadvantaged people to accept and thus benefit from universal services (Tudor Hart, 1971). Targeting is therefore believed to be more likely to reduce inequalities in health.

The case against targeting

On the other hand, there are several serious objections to targeting:

○ Targeting will benefit only a relatively small number of people as, by definition, only the high-risk tail of the distribution of risk is involved; by contrast, a universal approach can benefit much larger numbers at lower risk, reduces the numbers of those at highest risk by drawing the tail 'to the left' and reduces the chance of lower risk people drifting to the higher risk end of the distribution. This is a consequence of Rose's prevention paradox (Rose, 1981).

○ How can we know, a priori, who is at high risk? If defined in socio-economic terms, most of the population in some deprived communities will fall into this category. In the case of child development, socio-economic risk is too crude a tool for prediction of risk, and other methods have proven problematic. An analysis of data from a Scottish Government demonstration project ('Starting Well') data in Glasgow demonstrated that health visitors were unable to predict two-thirds of 'high-risk' families (in terms of future social service contacts) in families with children aged 0–4 months (Wright *et al.*, 2009).

○ Even if we can identify a high-risk group with sufficient accuracy, how can we predict, a priori, which individuals within the group will actually benefit from the intervention? High-risk groups may be most in need of services but least likely to benefit – the examples of heavy drinkers and smokers are often cited in this regard (see the last point in 'The case for targeting', above).

○ Targeting may carry a social stigma that creates a barrier to public acceptance, as has been repeatedly found in relation to publicly funded social welfare provision.

Conclusion

There are arguments for and against targeting. A combination of universal and targeted approaches, linked to evaluation, should remain the public health strategy of choice for injury prevention, as for other areas of public health.

◀LEARNING POINT▶

There are arguments for and against the targeting of high-risk groups in public health. A combination of universal and targeted approaches, linked to evaluation, should remain the public health strategy of choice for injury prevention as for other areas of public health.

Process of injury prevention policy development

The WHO (Schopper *et al.*, 2006, p. 4) has defined a policy (sometimes called a strategy or plan) as: 'a written document that provides the basis for action to be taken jointly by the government and its non-governmental partners.' When applied to injuries, Schopper *et al.* (2006, p. 5) extended this definition substantially: 'A policy on violence and injury prevention is a document that sets out the main principles and defines goals, objectives, prioritised actions and coordinated mechanisms, for preventing intentional and unintentional injuries and reducing their consequences.'

Although the WHO highlights the importance of policy development, equally vital are two further steps – implementation and evaluation. All three steps should be viewed as consistent with the public health approach ('diagnosis' – 'treatment' – 'follow-up') to injury prevention described earlier.

Rationale for an integrated approach to injury prevention policy-making

> Given the complex causality of violence and injuries, their prevention requires multisectoral and multidisciplinary efforts at national and local levels. (Sminkey, 2006)

By its nature, government is organised in vertical departments. This can result in a 'silo mentality' that is inefficient and obstructs progress. In the field of injury prevention, the following key national government agencies have remits and responsibilities that require to be taken into account in policy-making, implementation and evaluation:

- ❏ Health;
- ❏ Social services;
- ❏ Education;
- ❏ Justice;
- ❏ Housing;
- ❏ Transport;
- ❏ Environment;
- ❏ Industry.

Each sector has a specific role to play but may be unrelated to or unaware of the activities of the others. According to the WHO, health ministries should take the lead as injury is first and foremost a public health challenge. Whoever is the lead agency, some attempt is, however, necessary to achieve 'joined-up' policy development that will lead to the articulation of a single overarching policy statement setting out a common vision, strategies and objectives. The document should take the form of a policy, strategy or plan – depending on circumstances. That implies the application of a comprehensive approach that embraces all injury causes, types, severities and age groups. An integrated approach should help to:

- ❏ promote coherence;
- ❏ enhance synergies across sectors;
- ❏ identify gaps, conflicts, inconsistencies and duplication;
- ❏ allocate sufficient resources;
- ❏ increase visibility.

Few countries have such comprehensive policies for injury and violence prevention. Most policy statements focus only on a subtype of injury and emanate from a single sector, thereby rendering interagency collaboration less likely.

That WHO emphasises the unity of injuries by its use of the phrase 'injury and violence prevention' – despite its apparently tautological nature. It argues that a single policy that embraces all injuries is desirable on the following grounds:

- ❑ the greater potential for advocacy;
- ❑ the common data sets obtained from hospital surveillance and community surveys;
- ❑ the shared causal pathways (e.g. economic, social, environmental and behavioural);
- ❑ the frequent need for a multisectoral response (e.g. to alcohol misuse);
- ❑ the public health approach being common to all forms of injury prevention;
- ❑ the shared ethical considerations involved (e.g. social justice and equity);
- ❑ the 'final common pathway' of all injuries, i.e. the need for healthcare and rehabilitation.

To that list may be added a principle that is perhaps the most crucial of all: that countermeasures designed to prevent injuries are often the same whether the injury category is intentional or unintentional. One example is gun control that, if implemented effectively, will reduce the incidence of gunshot wounds whether inflicted intentionally or unintentionally. Another is action to reduce excessive alcohol consumption, as that substance is so frequently a trigger or risk factor for a wide range of injuries of multiple underlying aetiologies.

⌐LEARNING POINT

In developing policy, countermeasures designed to prevent injuries are often the same whether the injury category is intentional or unintentional.

The debate around integrated (horizontal) or focused (vertical) policy development can sometimes create a false dichotomy. These are not mutually exclusive positions. The decision to adopt a unitary, holistic approach to injury prevention does not preclude the parallel development of policies aimed at specific injury types or circumstances. On the contrary, such an approach may be regarded as complementary, synergistic and mutually reinforcing.

WHO guidelines for developing a policy response to injury

The WHO recommends that policies be developed in three phases:

- ❑ initiating the process;
- ❑ formulating the policy;
- ❑ seeking approval.

The timescale of these phases is difficult to predict, and there is likely to be some overlap.

Phase 1: Initiating the policy development process
This initial phase comprises four steps: assess the current situation, raise the level of awareness of the issues, identify leadership and nurture strong commitment, and finally involve all the key stakeholders. These four steps may be pursued either sequentially or simultaneously, depending on circumstances.

Step 1: Assess the situation
This is the 'diagnostic' step without which an appropriate 'treatment' in the form of a policy response is impossible. It comprises four elements: an epidemiological assessment (using routine or survey data); an intervention assessment (of what is already being done and what potential interventions are not being implemented for whatever reason); an assessment of existing policies (including laws, regulations and international conventions); and a stakeholder analysis (identification of all possible partners in government, industry, academia, the media and elsewhere, as well as possible opponents whose ultimate support may prove crucial).

Step 2: Raise awareness
The results from Step 1 should be used to mount a communication and lobbying exercise with a view to preparing public and political opinion for action. The basic premise should be that awareness is at a relatively low level among the general public, politicians, manufacturers, non-governmental organisations, community groups and other stakeholders. Media campaigns are often most effective when linked to nationally or internationally important days, events or festivals.

Step 3: Identify leadership and foster political commitment
Because policy development requires the cooperation of several government departments as well as non-governmental agencies, the process will only move forward if leadership is forthcoming. This is a formidable challenge. Large organisations are intrinsically inert, and a great deal of patience, persistence and persuasiveness is necessary to ensure that momentum is maintained. One way of achieving this is to set up a multisectoral steering group with the chairperson role rotating between all of the relevant departments.

Step 4: Involve stakeholders and create ownership
Securing stakeholder commitment to a new policy is so vital that it has to permeate every stage of the process. Apparently minor errors, such as forgetting to consult a key group or to include an organisation's logo on a document, can prove disastrous. Obtaining the goodwill and support of community groups is particularly important. There are various potential sources of tension here between the need for leadership on the one hand and stakeholder involvement on the other, or between the determination to drive an evidence-based but controversial policy through and the need to achieve a wide consensus.

■LEARNING POINT──────────────────────────────■

Securing stakeholder commitment to a new injury prevention policy is so vital that it has to permeate every stage of the policy development process.
● ●

Phase 2: Formulating the policy

Following initiation of the policy development process, the policy itself requires to be articulated. This task is usually assigned by the lead agency either to a designated individual or to a small group of professionals. This is a highly skilled undertaking, and the appropriate selection of the individuals or group is thus critical.

The document itself should be clearly written and well structured so that all of the sectors and stakeholders can understand it and how it relates to them. The WHO suggests taking three steps to writing such a document: define a framework, set objectives and select interventions, and ensure that policy leads to action.

Step 1: Define a framework for the policy document

Start by establishing a template for the overall shape and direction of the policy. Most successful policy documents include a simple, single, concise goal or 'vision' that indicates what the policy is supposed to achieve. These statements (e.g. 'securing safety for all' or 'towards an injury-free country') are, by their nature, idealistic, although it is sometimes helpful to indicate a timescale (e.g. 'a 5-year strategy'). The policy should be built upon explicit guiding principles to which stakeholders can relate. These might be general values (justice, equality, human rights) or explicit references to relevant national policies or international treaties.

Step 2: Set objectives and select interventions

This will probably comprise the main body of the document. More detailed objectives should elaborate upon the broad goals and be linked to means of achieving them. The WHO recommends a tiered approach to the statement of injury prevention objectives, broadly reflecting the need to reduce incidence, severity and consequences (primary, secondary and tertiary prevention). Such a systematic approach to objective-setting requires supportive data so that the effectiveness of the policy can monitored. These objectives are meaningless unless linked to a series of interventions for attaining them. The interventions should, as far as possible be evidence based, that is, drawn both from research and international experience, and should be presented in order of priority with estimated timescales for implementation.

Step 3: Ensure that policy leads to action

So far, the policy document amounts to little more than a statement of good intentions, however carefully crafted. To ensure that the policy is workable, several practical details will have to be addressed. These include setting priorities (which injuries will be addressed first), defining specific responsibilities (designating leadership and operational roles), describing resources and skills needed (finance and personnel), and creating mechanisms for monitoring and evaluation (of the process of policy development and its implementation).

Phase 3: Seeking approval and endorsement

The third and final phase in the policy development process reiterates elements of the earlier phases. The groundwork will have been prepared at a much earlier stage. In a sense, therefore, this phase merely reinforces and consolidates earlier achievements. The three components of this phase are the approval and endorsement of stakeholders, the government and the state (its parliament or legislature), respectively (although this process should be calibrated to match the prevailing political circumstances in a particular country or region). A consultative meeting to discuss a draft policy document is a well-tried means of securing stakeholder involvement, participation and endorsement. Once the text has been revised and approved by the consultees, the document can then be submitted to the relevant minister for approval by the cabinet or leader, and then by the parliament. This role is probably most efficiently undertaken by a nominated official or organisation within government to ensure that the process is negotiated smoothly.

These guidelines are intended to provide general pointers to effective policy development rather than being prescriptive instructions to be slavishly followed. In practice, many obstacles to progress are likely to appear that demand great flexibility, ingenuity and persistence on the part of professionals. Turning these guiding principles into action will form a key component of Section 2 of this book.

SUMMARY OF CHAPTER 3

Preventive approaches to injury

- The public health approach to a problem is analogous to the clinical triad of diagnosis, treatment and follow-up. It comprises three questions: what are the nature, scale, and determinants of the problem in the population ('diagnosis')?; what can and is being done to address it ('treatment')?; and how well are interventions being implemented and how might they be improved ('follow-up')?

- A specialised form of 'community diagnosis' in the injury prevention field is surveillance. Surveillance (or monitoring) is a form of routine statistical analysis of injury data that has been shown to be helpful in addressing the public health challenge of injury.

- The second step in the public health approach requires a distillation of the research evidence to identify efficacious interventions, combined with a review of what is actually being done in practice. Critical appraisal of the literature is the lynchpin of evidence-based practice.

- The third public health step demands an evaluation, audit or monitoring mechanism to determine the strengths and weaknesses of current interventions with a view to making recommendations for the future. This is probably the most neglected aspect of public health.

- Several studies have concluded that at least a third of all childhood injury deaths could be avoided were interventions of known efficacy implemented. Assessing the extent of this implementation gap is, however, difficult and controversial.

- Two of the most popular conceptual models of injury prevention are the three levels (primary, secondary, tertiary) of prevention and the three Es (education, enforcement and engineering/environment). Other useful models for injury prevention are Lalonde's health field concept, the social ecological model of Dahlgren and Krug, the Haddon Matrix and the WHO DPSEEA (drivers, pressures, states, exposures, effects, actions) sequence.

- Injury prevention should represent an outstanding financial investment. Unfortunately, the extent to which preventive measures generate long-term savings is uncertain as data are sparse and few cost–benefit analyses have been performed. Miller, using American data, has estimated that $7 is saved for every $1 invested in prevention.

- The WHO urges health ministries to take the lead in injury prevention as injury is a public health challenge. 'Joined-up' policy development is necessary to develop a single overarching policy statement setting out a common vision, strategies and objectives. The WHO recommends that policies be developed in three phases: initiating the process, formulating the policy, and seeking approval.

CHAPTER 4

Implementation and evaluation

Learning objectives

■ To be aware of the complex nature of the implementation of injury prevention policies
■ To understand the reasons for and elements of the evaluation of injury prevention
■ To be able to discuss why screening poses a special challenge for evaluation

Implementing injury prevention policies

Injury prevention policy-making at national level or regional level is a highly complex process (see Chapter 3). Even if the policy is sound and has been approved by all the relevant committees and stakeholders, it may never be implemented. Among the reasons for this are:

- ❑ lack of political commitment on the part of the relevant ministers or officials;
- ❑ inadequate protected funding for all stages of implementation;
- ❑ absence of expert advice on implementation;
- ❑ absence of delivery vehicles;
- ❑ inadequate resources, skills, training and research;
- ❑ disputes over the nature of monitoring and evaluation.

A striking example of a policy that was faultless in its conception, development and dissemination is the ill-fated report of the UK Task Force on Accidental Injury (Department of Health, 2002). This initiative appeared to have been largely driven by the effective lobbying of injury prevention professionals and researchers rather than by an explicit political decision. Furthermore, there were no clear lines of responsibility and accountability for the policy's implementation, nor were there mechanisms or vehicles for ensuring implementation within a given timescale. The end result was that the various recommendations, while sensible and uncontroversial, could not be carried through to implementation.

Some years later, many of the recommendations of the Task Force re-emerged in a different guise in the context of another policy initiative conducted by a different ministry – the Department for Children, Schools and Families (2008). The Staying Safe Action Plan actually went further than the Task Force report by integrating all aspects of injury prevention, including abuse and neglect, under the same policy rubric of 'safety promotion'. Whether or not by design, that formulation of the policy objective may have proved more politically acceptable and appealing to the wider public than the more technocratic term 'injury prevention'. New administrative structures – Safeguarding Children Boards – were created to translate the policy proposals into action, and clear guidelines were provided to these bodies to enable them to function efficiently and effectively.

What is evaluation?

As described earlier, evaluation is the public health analogy to the 'follow-up' component of clinical practice. The clinician needs to know how well the patient has responded to therapy; the public health practitioner needs to know the extent to which the target group or population has responded to the preventive intervention. Although it may seem self-evident that evaluation is important, and lip service is often paid to its inclusion by governments and agencies, reality frequently fails to match the rhetoric. This is because evaluation is easier to support in principle than to perform in practice. Evaluation is a component of the World Health Organisation's (WHO's) public health model of violence and injury prevention. Its purpose is to generate evidence about what works and monitor the effectiveness of intervention programmes, policies and measures.

The term 'evaluation' sounds scientific but it isn't. In essence, it means 'to determine the value of', but 'value' is a subjective concept. More formally, evaluation is defined as the 'systematic investigation of the merit, worth, or significance of an object' (paraphrased from Scriven, 1998). Evaluation in public health can be conducted in two distinct if interrelated ways (Figure 4.1). Evaluation undertaken in the context of research is useful in yielding information about what *can* work. This produces generalisable knowledge about *efficacy* – the extent to which an intervention has been shown to work in ideal or experimental conditions. This kind of evaluation is sometimes distinguished from investigations that assess the extent to which interventions actually work in practice. The context of the latter is usually a service

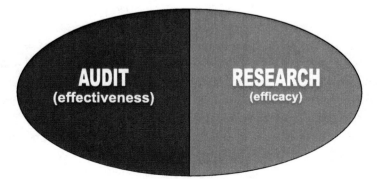

Figure 4.1 Two types of evaluation for audit or research.

or programme, and it produces non-generalisable information about *effectiveness*. Synonyms for this type of evaluation include monitoring, programme review or audit.

LEARNING POINT

The term evaluation sounds scientific but it isn't. In essence, it means 'to determine the value of', but 'value' is a subjective concept.

The generally accepted or gold standard method for generating evidence arising from the evaluation of efficacy is the meta-analysis or systematic review. Lower down the hierarchy of evidence come at least one large, well-conducted randomised controlled trial, non-randomised controlled experiments, before-and-after studies (with or without control groups) and finally 'expert opinion'. Most non-research types of evaluation will have to operate lower rather than higher in the hierarchy.

The context of programme, service or policy evaluation is the *planning cycle* – what are the objectives of the programme, service or policy, how are they being met, what are the results? So evaluation should be linked – like audit – into the planning cycle.

Programme or policy evaluation is sometimes subdivided into two subtypes – formative and summative. A formative evaluation is undertaken during the development of a programme, enabling changes to be made in either its objectives or its implementation. This type of evaluation frequently focuses on staff or participant attitudes, performance or satisfaction. A summative evaluation usually comes later in the process and is designed to provide insights into the effectiveness of a programme over a defined period of time; it is useful in deciding whether to continue, expand or terminate an established programme.

Evaluation is often constructed theoretically in relation to objectives across the three dimensions of structure–process–outcome (Donabedian, 2003), although sometimes 'impact' is preferred to or is added to outcome. These terms are largely self-explanatory, but the selection of appropriate indicators can be highly problematic and constrained by the accessibility and quality of the available data.

> **Box 4.1 Evaluation of injury prevention measures – guidelines for professionals using the five-step evaluation model**
> (Based on a presentation by Dahlberg and Stone entitled 'Outcome evaluation' at the WHO Third Milestones of a Global Campaign of Violence Prevention Meeting, Scotland, 2007.)
>
> **Step 1: Clarify programme goals/objectives**
>
> **What is a goal? It is a general statement about what you are trying to achieve. Objectives indicate how the goal will be achieved (N.B. Objectives should be SMART – specific, measurable, action-oriented, realistic and time-specific)**

Step 2: Design an evaluation plan
- ✔ Decide who is your target audience
- ✔ Clarify the timescale and resources
- ✔ Select an evaluation framework (e.g. structure–process–outcome)
- ✔ Choose an appropriate evaluation method

Step 3: Develop and implement a data collection plan
- ✔ Decide whether to collect quantitative or qualitative data – or both
- ✔ Choose specific types of data to collect (e.g. demographic, mortality, self-report or observational)
- ✔ Collect the data

Step 4: Analyse and interpret the data
- ✔ Prepare the data for analysis
- ✔ Analyse the data
- ✔ Interpret the results

Step 5: Use and report your findings
- ✔ Select your audience (e.g. policy, academic) depending on purpose)
- ✔ Present your findings in an appropriate format
- ✔ Recommend – where necessary – changes to the programme

In practice, it does not usually matter which particular evaluation method is used. A key dual message is that evaluation is worthwhile although challenging and that outcome evaluation should not be conducted on its own. We need to know about both the objectives and the process because this information is essential to understanding what went right or what went wrong.

■ LEARNING POINT ────────────────────────────────────

The five steps of evaluation in injury prevention are: clarify the objectives; design an evaluation plan; develop a data collection plan; analyse and interpret the data; and use and report your findings.
• •

The special case of screening

All forms of public health intervention should be subjected to evaluation, audit or monitoring, and these general principles of evaluation are widely applicable. Nevertheless, there are some circumstances in which special evaluation principles or criteria have been developed. One of these is screening or early detection through mass testing. Screening has been one of the lynchpins of public health since the mid-20th century and has been surrounded by controversy for most of its history.

The UK National Screening Committee has defined screening as follows:

> Screening is a process of identifying apparently healthy people who may be at increased risk of a disease or condition. They can then be offered

information, further tests and appropriate treatment to reduce their risk and/or any complications arising from the disease or condition. (www. screening.nhs.uk/criteria accessed 7 February 2011)

Screening is sometimes relevant to injury prevention. It may be advocated for the early identification and avoidance of risk factors (e.g. alcohol misuse or severe deprivation), for the detection of signs of injury (e.g. abuse or neglect in children) that require special clinical or social interventions, and for the early diagnosis of important and potentially debilitating sequelae of injuries (e.g. post-traumatic stress disorder).

Screening is a seductive idea as it appears to be based on the unarguable premise that early diagnosis equals better prognosis. In practice, however, the premise turns out to be flawed: not only does screening fail to improve outcomes in many cases, but it may also actually cause harm by generating anxiety, additional work and expense, and producing side effects and complications of unnecessary diagnostic or therapeutic procedures. Injury prevention practitioners and policy-makers should be aware of the possibilities and pitfalls of screening.

In 1968, at the request of the WHO, Wilson and Jungner (1968) set out a set of principles that drew attention to the need to reflect carefully on the pros and cons of screening prior to the implementation of a programme. These have stood the test of time well, although the UK National Screening Committee subsequently refined and elaborated on them.

UK National Screening Committee Criteria for appraising the viability, effectiveness and appropriateness of a screening programme

Ideally, all the following criteria should be met before screening is initiated.

The condition

- ❏ The condition should be an important health problem.
- ❏ The epidemiology and natural history of the condition, including development from latent to declared disease, should be adequately understood, and there should be a detectable risk factor, disease marker, latent period or early symptomatic stage.
- ❏ All the cost-effective primary prevention interventions should have been implemented as far as is practicable.
- ❏ If the carriers of a mutation are identified as a result of screening, the natural history of people with this status should be understood, including the psychological implications.

The test

- ❏ There should be a simple, safe, precise and validated screening test.
- ❏ The distribution of test values in the target population should be known and a suitable cut-off level defined and agreed.
- ❏ The test should be acceptable to the population.

❑ There should be an agreed policy on the further diagnostic investigation of individuals with a positive test result and on the choices available to those individuals.

❑ If the test is for mutations, the criteria used to select the subset of mutations to be covered by screening, if all possible mutations are not being tested, should be clearly set out.

The treatment

❑ There should be an effective treatment or intervention for patients identified through early detection, with evidence of early treatment leading to better outcomes than late treatment.

❑ There should be agreed evidence-based policies covering which individuals should be offered treatment and the appropriate treatment to be offered.

❑ Clinical management of the condition and patient outcomes should be optimised in all healthcare providers prior to participation in a screening programme.

The screening programme

❑ There should be evidence from high-quality randomised controlled trials that the screening programme is effective in reducing mortality or morbidity. Where screening is aimed solely at providing information to allow the person being screened to make an 'informed choice' (e.g. Down syndrome or cystic fibrosis carrier screening), there must be evidence from high-quality trials that the test accurately measures risk. The information that is provided about the test and its outcome must be of value and readily understood by the individual being screened.

❑ There should be evidence that the complete screening programme (test, diagnostic procedures and treatment/intervention) is clinically, socially and ethically acceptable to health professionals and the public.

❑ The benefit from the screening programme should outweigh the physical and psychological harm (caused by the test, diagnostic procedures and treatment).

❑ The opportunity cost of the screening programme (including testing, diagnosis and treatment, administration, training and quality assurance) should be economically balanced in relation to expenditure on medical care as a whole (i.e. value for money). Assessment against these criteria should have regard to evidence from cost–benefit and/or cost-effectiveness analyses and have regard to the effective use of available resource.

❑ All other options for managing the condition (e.g. improving treatment or providing other services) should have been considered to ensure that no more cost-effective intervention could be introduced or current interventions increased within the resources available.

- ❏ There should be a plan for managing and monitoring the screening programme and an agreed set of quality assurance standards.
- ❏ Adequate staffing and facilities for testing, diagnosis, treatment and programme management should be available prior to the commencement of the screening programme.
- ❏ Evidence-based information, explaining the consequences of testing, investigation and treatment, should be made available to potential participants to assist them in making an informed choice.
- ❏ Public pressure for widening the eligibility criteria or reducing the screening interval, and for increasing the sensitivity of the testing process, should be anticipated. Decisions about these parameters should be scientifically justifiable to the public.
- ❏ If screening is for a mutation, the programme should be acceptable to people identified as carriers and to other family members.

Why is screening considered a special case for evaluation? After all, identifying a disorder earlier rather than later seems a relatively innocuous idea to which most sensible people would subscribe. On closer examination, however, screening turns out to be much more complex an activity than it first appears. Take conventional clinical care: a patient with a problem approaches the health service for advice and, where appropriate, treatment, and the service responds with no prior promise of success. Screening, by contrast, is offered to people who have not usually sought help. In other words, it is undertaken at the initiative of the service rather than the patient. The implication is that screening will confer some benefit, otherwise it would not be offered to the public. That obliges the screening providers to be reasonably confident that the screening programme will benefit those screened.

These unusual characteristics of screening that have been translated into principles or criteria for the purposes either of considering whether or not to implement a screening programme, or of evaluating an established one, or both. These concerns may be grouped under three headings: ethical, scientific and economic.

The *ethical* criteria include the following: it should be demonstrated that the problem is an important one from a public health perspective; the screening test should reach the population at risk; the screening test must be acceptable to the subjects; effective treatment should be available should screening reveal a disorder; and the benefits of screening should be known to outweigh the harm.

The *scientific* criteria include that: the natural history (including the preclinical time span) of the disorder should be understood; the validity of the screening (sensitivity and specificity) should be known; and a clear consensus on what constitutes a positive test result should exist.

The *economic* criteria encompass: that there should be an understanding of the resource requirements of screening and the subsequent investigations and follow-up;

that the economic costs and benefits should be known, with the latter outweighing the former; and that the opportunity costs (i.e. the costs of diverting resources away from other activities towards screening) should be estimated.

These special principles of screening have a common theme: all public health professionals should be aware of the need to challenge the widespread assumption, often based on inadequate evidence, that the earlier detection of a disorder or risk factor through screening is bound to be beneficial. Although there are some examples of highly successful screening (e.g. for neonatal disorders such as hypothyroidism or for coronary heart disease risk factors in middle-aged adults), the reality is that the claims for screening are often exaggerated.

◀ LEARNING POINT ▶ ━━━━━━━━━━━━━━━━━━━━━━━━━━━━

All practitioners should be aware of the need to challenge the widespread assumption, often based on inadequate evidence, that the earlier detection of a disorder or risk factor through screening is bound to be beneficial.
• •

Concluding observations on evaluation: some pitfalls

There is often a huge gap between the theory and practice of evaluation. Much of the rhetoric about evaluation is unrealistic and is used as a fig leaf to push through controversial interventions. Being aware of some of the most common practical pitfalls confronting practitioners and policy-makers should help in their avoidance.

There may be confusion about the purpose of an evaluation study. This often revolves around whether new knowledge is being generated or a service is being audited or monitored. In the former case, a randomised controlled trial is the gold standard experimental method, with controlled observational studies occupying the runner-up position. In the latter case, an uncontrolled observation over time may be sufficient. Clarification of the purpose of the exercise is essential at the outset. The key question to be addressed is this: is the evaluation intended to generate new, generalisable knowledge about the efficacy of the intervention or programme, or is its purpose to assess the effectiveness of an intervention or programme in a particular time and place?

Feelings often run high about evaluation – perhaps because value judgements are inevitably involved. There is often a gulf of understanding between researchers, who see evaluation as a methodologically rigorous approach that should assist the successful implementation and refinement of an intervention, and practitioners, who may regard it, at best, as excessively reliant on irrelevant 'academic theory' or, at worst, as a criticism of or a threat to their professional integrity or competence.

Learning lessons from evaluation may be a painful process but should be welcomed. Outcome indicators may be contentious and deemed either inappropriate or immeasurable. The results of an evaluation may be negative or ambiguous for methodological reasons (e.g. too small a sample size or low quality of the data collected) that produce a misleading picture. And an expected outcome may not be achieved either because the intervention was ineffective or because the intervention was poorly implemented.

Evaluation can be internal or external. The former is more practical, while the latter is more objective. Ideally, a combination of both should be used. Restricting evaluation to an internal exercise, in which the participants have a vested interest, may be tempting to the programme managers but will seriously damage the credibility of the findings.

◄ LEARNING POINT

Evaluation can be internal or external. The former is more practical, while the latter is more objective. Ideally, a combination of both should be used.

Absence of evidence is not the same as evidence of absence of efficacy. Public health professionals always have to apply an element of judgement in deciding whether or not to proceed with a particular policy or practice, regardless of scientific considerations, while taking account of the evidence. The way this professional judgement has been conceptualised in clinical practice has been enormously influential in the public health field and will be described in greater detail in the next chapter.

SUMMARY OF CHAPTER 4

Implementation and evaluation

- Injury prevention policy-making is a highly complex process. Even if the policy is sound and has been approved by all the relevant committees and stakeholders, it may never be implemented.

- Failure to implement injury prevention policy is attributable to several recurring obstacles: lack of political commitment from the relevant ministers or officials; inadequate protected funding for all stages of implementation; absence of expert advice on implementation; absence of delivery vehicles; inadequate resources, skills, training and research; and disputes over the nature of monitoring and evaluation.

- While it may seem self-evident that evaluation is important, and lip service is often paid to its inclusion by governments and agencies, reality frequently fails to match the rhetoric. This is because evaluation is easier to support in principle than to perform in practice.

- Evaluation undertaken in the context of research is useful in yielding information about what can work (efficacy); this kind of evaluation is sometimes distinguished from investigations that assess what does work (effectiveness). Synonyms for the latter form of evaluation include monitoring, programme review and audit.

- The gold standard method for generating evidence arising from evaluation is the meta-analysis or systematic review of randomised controlled trials. Lower down the hierarchy of evidence come at least one large, well-conducted randomised controlled trial, non-randomised controlled experiments, before-and-after studies and finally 'expert opinion'. Most non-research types of evaluation will have to operate lower rather than higher in the hierarchy.

■ Evaluation is often constructed theoretically in relation to objectives across the three dimensions of structure–process–outcome (or sometimes 'impact'). These terms are largely self-explanatory, but the selection of appropriate indicators can be highly problematic and constrained by the accessibility and quality of the available data.

■ Screening is sometimes relevant to injury prevention. It may be advocated for the early identification and avoidance of risk factors, for the detection of signs of injury that require special clinical or social interventions, and for the early diagnosis of potentially debilitating sequelae of injuries. Screening should be subjected to a specialised form of evaluation because of the unique ethical concerns relating to it.

■ Absence of evidence of efficacy is not the same as evidence of absence of efficacy. Public health professionals have to apply judgement in deciding whether or not to proceed with a particular policy or practice.

SECTION 2

PRACTICE OF INJURY PREVENTION

Section 2 Overview

This section applies the principles described in Section 1 in a way that demonstrates how the main players can translate theory into practice using the best available evidence. It comprises four chapters and their summaries:

5. From theory to practice

6. Implementing unintentional injury prevention

7. Implementing intentional injury prevention

8. Combined public health and clinical approaches

CHAPTER 5

From theory to practice

Learning objectives

- To be aware of some of the major obstacles to translating injury prevention principles into practice
- To have a knowledge of the principles of evidence-based public health practice
- To understand the nature of evidence-based injury prevention – assessing the evidence base, applying professional judgement, and involving the public

Obstacles to translating injury prevention principles into practice

Injury prevention policy and practice is easier to talk about than to implement. As in other areas of public health, the road from theory to practice can be a long and winding one punctuated by numerous potential pitfalls. Translating research into practice is particularly challenging. A novel English experiment (Kelly *et al.*, 2004; Brussoni *et al.*, 2006), whereby evidence briefings were presented and discussed at a series of joint meetings of researchers and practitioners until consensus was achieved, illustrates one possible solution. In a commentary on that paper, US writers (Mallonee *et al.*, 2006) asserted that behavioural factors, notably the 'enthusiasm, skills and cultural competence' of the practitioner, were key ingredients of success.

All injury prevention begins with a rather abstract idea or vision that then evolves, often in fits and starts, into a plan, strategy, policy, programme or initiative. Ensuring that evidence-based aspirations reach fruition depends on a range of factors, some of which will lie outside of the practitioner's control. Nevertheless, many obstacles are highly predictable. Here is a list of some of these, along with their implications for the practitioner:

Much ignorance, indifference and prejudice about the subject has to be overcome. The 'accidents will happen' mentality remains ubiquitous both among the general public and practitioners.
Implication: Prepare the ground by ensuring that stakeholders appreciate the underlying philosophical premise of injury prevention – that injuries are predictable and avoidable. Do not take this premise for granted as some people do not subscribe to

it despite the wealth of research evidence in its favour. A potentially effective means of overcoming this obstacle is to select, distribute and discuss a published statement issued by the World Health Organization (WHO), an injury professional lobby group or a prestigious journal.

Agreement on the basic concepts, definitions, terminology and classification systems relating to injury can be elusive.
Implication: Write a brief statement of what you mean by an injury, what terminology you are using and how you wish to classify injuries. Reference to an internationally agreed publication, such as the International Classification of Diseases (Tenth Revision), or the International Classification of External Causes of Injury, may be helpful.

Available routine data, on the incidence, circumstances, severity and outcomes of injury in a population, are often absent or inadequate for prevention.
Implication: Identify and list the various data sources, along with their main strengths and weaknesses, that you propose drawing upon to estimate need. These may include mortality, emergency department attendances and hospital discharge or survey data that are relevant to the population under scrutiny.

High-quality research studies on injury epidemiology, natural history, consequences and costs are relatively few in number and may be mutually contradictory.
Implication: Summarise – drawing on published systematic literature reviews where possible – some selected insights from the global literature on the particular injuries that you are addressing, indicating where knowledge is absent. Keep this very brief, using bullet points or diagrams to underline your main messages.

Identifying a robust evidence base for planning interventions demands a sophisticated level of understanding of research data and a high level of critical appraisal skills that are extremely rare.
Implication: Outline your approach to the critical appraisal of the research literature, or identify an academic collaborator with the appropriate skills. An effective short cut is to rely upon published summaries of research evidence from specialised groups such as the Cochrane Collaboration, the UK National Institute for Health and Clinical Excellence, the WHO or other sources of policy and practice guidance.

Securing strong and sustained professional and political commitment to injury prevention, beyond vague strategic aspirations, is difficult in the face of many competing demands.
Implication: Forge a link with one or more senior policy-makers and maintain consistent communication with them or their staff. Be opportunistic by highlighting injury issues currently receiving media attention. Avoid strident or hectoring

language, and always approach policy-makers in a spirit of constructive support rather than critical challenge.

Translating policies or strategies into practice may be problematic due to an absence of stakeholder involvement, adequate resources, skills, vehicles for delivery, managerial oversight and careful monitoring.

Implication: As far as possible, anticipate and try to address the need to involve stakeholders early, secure adequate resources, make use of academic and professional expertise, design vehicles for effective and efficient implementation, institute managerial oversight and introduce a mechanism for monitoring progress.

Early enthusiasm may dissipate due to changing personnel, nebulous objectives, disappointing or ambiguous outcomes, and interagency or interprofessional rivalry.

Implication: Reinforce staff motivation regularly through face-to-face contacts, newsletters, briefing meetings and progress reports. Ensure objectives are articulated clearly, acknowledge the absence of unequivocally positive outcomes, and try to mediate between professionals or agencies in a non-partisan manner.

Evaluation, when it is performed at all, may focus on process rather than outcomes, and operate over too short a time span to be able to demonstrate significant results.

Implication: Incorporate a framework for evaluation into the objectives and seek to measure progress in terms of both processes and outcomes over a sufficient period of time. Argue the case for extra resources to be devoted exclusively to evaluation as a means of raising the profile of the initiative and enhancing the reputation of the agency and its personnel.

Public opinion is fickle and may quickly shift away from support for unobtrusive and low-key prevention back towards dramatic and highly visible acute trauma care.

Implication: Include a communications strategy in any new preventive initiative and recruit, where necessary, professional help to implement it. Offer to give media interviews (or to nominate an appropriately skilled individual), and issue regular press releases that focus on the importance and achievements of preventive measures.

Practising evidence-based injury prevention

In identifying and implementing injury prevention measures, practitioners are coming under increasing pressure to justify their decisions in terms of the published research evidence. The intention is clear and laudable – to expend time, energy and resources on measures that are likely to yield real benefits to the population. An evidence-based approach has become de rigueur. Yet there is a common misconception about 'evidence-based' public health. As with evidence-based clinical practice, an evidence-based approach does not mean that the practitioner is required to suspend professional judgement and slavishly adopt guidelines based on robust research. What is the 'evidence-based' approach?

■(LEARNING POINT)────────────────────────────

An evidence-based approach does not mean that the practitioner is required to suspend professional judgement and slavishly adopt guidelines based on robust research. Two other dimensions are involved: the judgement of the professional and the perspective of the target population.
● ●

The pioneers of evidence-based medical practice (notably Sackett and his colleagues at McMaster University in Canada) advocated the use of good quality research studies, mainly in the form of randomised controlled trials (RCTs), as the foundation for medical practice.

Sackett and Straus (1998, p. 1336) defined evidence-based medicine as 'the integration of best research evidence with clinical expertise and patient values'. Much initial resistance to the ideas of Sackett and his colleagues was rooted in a fear of 'recipe book medicine' in which hard-won clinical skills would be marginalised. The authors' intention, however, was not to undermine clinical judgement but to improve it through reference to relevant research. Moreover, they argued that a third component was necessary – the perspective of the patient. This led to the development of a triangulation process (Figure 5.1) whereby the perspectives of

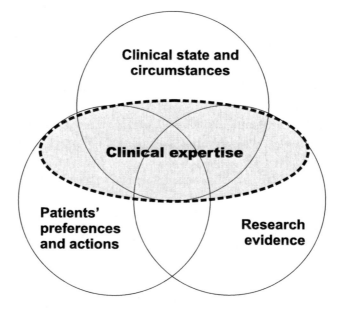

Figure 5.1 The evidence-based practice triangle. After Sackett *et al.* (2000).

the doctor and the patient, supplemented by the insights generated by appropriate research, would combine in a way that enhanced clinical skill and improved clinical outcomes.

Evidence-based public health policy and practice reflects this clinical approach. It comprises a similar process of triangulation that incorporates an assessment of scientific evidence, the judgement of the professional and the perspective of the target population (the 'patient').

Assessing the evidence

The rapid rise in the number of public health research papers in the last half-century is both a blessing and a curse. A growing evidence base can only help professional decision-making about which measures and programmes are brought to bear on a particular public health challenge. On the other hand, however, the sheer volume of data has become so overwhelming that no one individual can possibly absorb it in a manner that facilitates rational decision-making. That has let to the development of the twin concepts of critical appraisal and systematic reviews, whereby a large body of published literature may be distilled down, by specialist researchers, to its essential, bottom-line messages.

Critical appraisal is the process of systematically assessing research reports to judge their trustworthiness, value and relevance in a particular context. Critical appraisal has greatly helped in the prioritisation of research findings into a hierarchy of evidence. Typically, this is characterised as ranging from expert opinion (the lowest level of evidence) to systematic reviews and meta-analyses (the highest level of evidence). Occupying an intermediate status in this evidence hierarchy are RCTs, of which there are relatively few in the injury prevention field compared with, say, cancer therapy. The interpretation and summarising of research evidence in this way has become increasingly sophisticated and standardised through the efforts of specialised researchers associated with initiatives such as the Cochrane Collaboration. The end point of this type of activity is usually the development of practice or policy guidelines, thereby opening up a channel of communication between researchers and practitioners.

■─(LEARNING POINT)─────────────────────────────

Critical appraisal of scientific papers has helped in the prioritisation of research findings into a hierarchy of evidence that ranges from expert opinion (the lowest level of evidence) to systematic reviews and meta-analyses (the highest level of evidence).

Professional judgement

Research evidence does not exist in a vacuum. It needs to be evaluated by professionals who must then decide what action to take based upon their understanding of that evidence. And the defining characteristic of any professional is the capacity to exert independent professional judgement that derives from the acquisition of skills during a recognised and documented training process.

Eraut (1994) describes professional judgement as 'that mysterious quality' nvolving the *terpretative* use of knowledge, practical w dom, a sense of purpose, appropriateness and feasibility. The key phrase is 'the interpretative use of knowledge' and implies that research evidence must be placed in a wider context. Professional judgement is especially crucial when the research evidence is absent, ambiguous or controversial. A purist academic posture is liable to prove unhelpful or even counterproductive.

What is often forgotten is that not all preventive measures need to be based on RCTs; those RCTs may not have been performed for good reasons. RCTs are only necessary when there is *equipoise* between two (or more) alternatives – that is, a controversy or question about which of the competing alternatives should be endorsed. And not all promising research findings should be instantly translated into action without taking account of the wider, social, political and economic implications.

◀ LEARNING POINT ▶

RCTs are only necessary when there is *equipoise* between two (or more) alternatives – that is, a controversy or question about which of the competing alternatives should be endorsed.

Involving the public

At one time, there was a common belief that large sections of the general public, particularly in disadvantaged communities, were either unaware of or uninformed about safety matters. That view led to an excessive and, as it transpired, misplaced reliance on educational campaigns to banish this ignorance. Empirical qualitative research carried out on a relatively poor urban estate in Glasgow (Roberts *et al.*, 1995) demonstrated the opposite: people were acutely aware of the dangers posed to their children but felt powerless to take the necessary preventive action. Moreover, when asked, they were enthusiastic advocates of safety measures and were willing to offer innovative ideas for their implementation. Since then, this phenomenon has been reported from around the world, notably through surveys undertaken in the context of the WHO's Safe Communities Network. Even relatively young children have been found to form a remarkably sophisticated view of safety and how it might be promoted.

A survey of a fairly small sample children and young people was commissioned by the Scottish Child Safety Alliance (Royal Society for the Prevention of Accidents/ Child Accident Prevention Trust, 2007) to elicit their views on unintentional injuries and their prevention, and to produce a snapshot of their risk-taking behaviour. The survey, which was undertaken by Children in Scotland, included online and printed questionnaires. The survey reported the following:

- ❏ Children and young people were worried about being injured in an accident.
- ❏ Having personal experience or personal knowledge of an unintentional injury requiring hospitalisation did not necessarily modify behaviour.
- ❏ A high proportion of children and young people either thought they already knew all they needed to know to stay safe, or rejected the whole idea that accidents can be prevented.
- ❏ A significant percentage of respondents admitted often engaging in behaviours that they knew could result in injury serious enough to require at least an overnight stay in hospital.
- ❏ The uptake of seat belt wearing was high, and knowledge of where to go and what to do in the event of a fire was good.
- ❏ Some respondents wanted to learn more about accident prevention and showed a marked willingness to take real responsibility for keeping themselves safe.

The UK National Health Service (NHS) asserts that it is fully committed to 'public involvement' in a way that goes beyond consulting patients either individually or in groups. The phrase smacks of political correctness, but that would be to misjudge it. Indeed, public involvement has become enshrined in legislation on the way the NHS operates. Here is a typical statement of that commitment from the Department of Health:

> Commissioners act on behalf of the public and patients. They are responsible for investing funds on behalf of their communities, and building local trust and legitimacy through the process of engagement with their local population. In order to make commissioning decisions that reflect the needs, priorities and aspirations of the local population, world class commissioners will engage with the public, and actively seek the views of patients, carers and the wider community. This new relationship with the public is long term, inclusive and enduring, and has been forged through a sustained effort and commitment on the part of commissioners. Decisions are made with a strong mandate from the local population and other partners.
> (www.dh.gov.uk/prod_consum_dh/groups/dh_digitalassets/documents/digitalasset/dh_080952.pdf accessed 25 February 2011)

These three components of an evidence-based approach – assessing the evidence, professional judgement and involving the public – are equally important in all forms of public health practice. All should be considered when planning an injury prevention intervention or policy, although it may not always prove possible to invoke all of them to the same degree.

Similarly, evidence-based injury prevention relies on these three components. Identifying the evidence base on which to base decisions about interventions is probably the easiest of the three.

SUMMARY OF CHAPTER 5

From theory to practice

- All injury prevention begins with an abstract idea or vision that then evolves into a plan, strategy, policy, programme or initiative. Ensuring that evidence-based aspirations reach fruition depends on a range of factors, some of which lie outside of the practitioner's control.

- As with evidence-based clinical practice, an evidence-based public health approach does not require practitioners to suspend professional judgement and slavishly adopt guidelines based on research.

- Evidence-based practice involves a triangulation process whereby the perspectives of the doctor and the patient, supplemented by the insights generated by appropriate research, combine in a way that enhances clinical skill and improves clinical outcomes.

- The three components of an evidence-based approach – assessing the evidence, professional judgement and involving the public – are equally important in all forms of public health practice. All should be considered when planning an injury prevention intervention or policy, although it may not always prove possible to invoke all of them to the same degree.

- Research evidence, although important, must be placed in a wider context. Professional judgement is especially crucial when the research evidence is absent, ambiguous or controversial. A purist academic posture is liable to prove unhelpful or even counterproductive.

- Not all preventive measures need to be based on knowledge derived from RCTs. Those RCTs may not have been performed for good reasons. RCTs are only necessary when there is equipoise between two (or more) alternatives – that is, a controversy or question about which of the competing alternatives should be endorsed.

- In the past, there was a common and mistaken belief that large sections of the general public were either unaware of or uninformed about safety matters. This view led to an excessive and misplaced reliance on educational campaigns to banish this supposed ignorance.

- Empirical research demonstrates that people are acutely aware of the dangers posed to their children but may feel powerless to take the necessary preventive action. Moreover, when asked, they are often enthusiastic advocates of safety measures and are willing to offer innovative ideas for their implementation.

- Research has shown that children and young people worry about being injured, although they may think they already know enough to stay safe, or may reject the whole idea that injuries can be prevented. Some show a marked willingness to take real responsibility for keeping themselves safe.

CHAPTER 6

Implementing unintentional injury prevention

Learning objectives

- To have a basic knowledge of the research evidence on the efficacy of unintentional injury prevention interventions
- To be aware of some of the key sources of guidance on child injury prevention
- To be able to describe the key measures that appear to be efficacious in unintentional child injury prevention

Outline of research evidence on the efficacy of interventions

As explained earlier, all preventive measures are nowadays expected to conform to principles of evidence-based practice, notably the integration of research findings and public perception with professional judgement. This in turn depends on the availability of robust research findings. The development and evaluation of injury prevention measures has been somewhat neglected by public health researchers, but that scenario appears to be changing. The evidence base for the efficacy of injury prevention has expanded substantially in recent years. This provides a solid foundation on which practitioners and policy-makers can plan and implement injury prevention measures.

In recent years, there have been numerous research studies, reviews, guidelines and other texts that, taken together, offer practitioners and policy-makers a formidable array of resources on which to draw for the purpose of implementing evidence-based injury prevention measures. Much of this material is now available electronically through specialised websites and Internet search engines. This explosion of knowledge is a double-edged sword. On the one hand, globally generated information has never been more voluminous or accessible; on the other hand, it can be overwhelming and indigestible. As a comprehensive account of all this material is virtually impossible within one book, the author has been deliberately selective in attempting to offer readers useful guidance in the form of a synthesis drawn from a relatively small number of authoritative sources.

Selected sources of guidance on child injury prevention

The evidence presented below has been derived and distilled from multiple and overlapping sources including the UK's Department of Health (2002) and National Institute for Health and Clinical Excellence (2010), EuroSafe (Mackay *et al.*, 2006), and the World Health Organization (WHO; Peden *et al.*, 2008).

Recommendations of the UK Accidental Injury Task Force 2000–2

In the late 1990s, the UK Government committed itself to injury prevention. A 1999 public health White Paper set national targets for the reduction in injury death rates (by at least one-fifth) and serious injury rates (by at least one-tenth) in England by 2010.

Taking its cue from the White Paper, the Department of Health subsequently established a multidisciplinary Accidental Injury Task Force (AITF) in 2000. Its remit was to advise the Chief Medical Officer for England on the most important priorities for action to prevent unintentional injuries in the population. As described earlier, its report (Department of Health, 2002) contained several recommendations relating directly to children. The AITF identified two vulnerable population groups for priority attention – young people (children and young adults) and older people. Two parallel working groups were set up to consider what action was needed to protect these groups from accidental injury. They concluded that much could be done to address the major causes of injury – namely falls, road casualties and dwelling fires – across all age groups. Their specific preventive recommendations (not elaborated here) were evidence-based although filtered through the sometimes divergent views of researchers, practitioners and civil servants.

The AITF also identified the following 10 steps to help deliver successful local implementation:

1. Use data collected in a common format to show where action is needed most.
2. Adapt key interventions to specific local needs where they will have the greatest impact.
3. Develop and disseminate good practice to show what can be done.
4. Show how these interventions can help deliver other programmes and meet targets elsewhere.
5. Involve all stakeholders in producing a local action plan.
6. Develop a well-trained workforce with the capacity to undertake injury prevention work.
7. Recruit high-level support.
8. Recruit support from the voluntary sector.
9. Identify sources of additional funding.
10. Identify indicators to monitor performance.

The AITF recommendations were never fully implemented, but many of them remain valid today.

The European Child Safety Good Practice Guide

Later publications from international sources, notably the European Child Safety Alliance (ECSA) of EuroSafe, have reinforced and expanded the AITF's recommendations. The ECSA team (Mackay *et al.*, 2006) attempted to integrate systematic reviews of evaluational research with expert views in an effort to describe 'good practice'. This philosophy fits well with the evidence-based approach described earlier. More precisely, the authors adopted the following definition of good practice:

- ❏ A prevention strategy that has been evaluated and found to be effective (either through systematic review or at least one rigorous evaluation) OR
- ❏ A prevention strategy where rigorous evaluation is difficult but expert opinion supports the practice and data suggest it is an effective strategy OR
- ❏ A prevention strategy where rigorous evaluation is difficult but expert opinion supports the practice and there is a clear link between the strategy and reduced risk but a less clear link between the strategy and reduced injuries AND
- ❏ The strategy in question has been implemented in a real world setting so that the practicality of the intervention has also been examined.

The findings of this analysis of the efficacy of interventions are fairly similar to those of the AITF (Department of Health, 2002), and the more recent reports from WHO (Peden *et al.*, 2008).

WHO European and World Reports on Child Injury Prevention

These two complementary documents adopt, as expected, a similar perspective rooted in the WHO's firm commitment to a public health approach to injury prevention.

The European report (Sethi *et al.*, 2008) asserts that where countries have shifted from trying to change individual behaviour to providing safe environments, they have reduced fatalities and health inequalities. The report identifies a series of strategic action points and proposes a number of effective interventions.

━◖LEARNING POINT◗━━━━━━━━━━━━━━━━━━━━━━━

Where countries have shifted from trying to change individual behaviour to providing safe environments, they have reduced fatalities and health inequalities.

The nine strategic action points are as follows:

- ❏ Integrate child injury prevention into a comprehensive approach to child and adolescent health.
- ❏ Develop and implement a child injury prevention plan involving other sectors.

❑ Implement evidence-based actions to prevent and control childhood injuries.

❑ Strengthen health systems to address child injuries.

❑ Build capacity and exchange best practice.

❑ Enhance the quality and quantity of data for child injury prevention.

❑ Support research and evaluation on the causes, consequences, costs and prevention of child injuries.

❑ Raise awareness and target investments for child injury prevention.

❑ Address inequity in child injury.

The WHO *World Report on Child Injury Prevention* (Peden *et al.*, 2008) is rather more topic focused and emphasises the need to take account of the limited resources available to low-income countries that together contribute the vast majority of child injury deaths in the world. The starting point of the report is the epidemiological burden of each group of injuries. Contributors were asked to formulate recommendations based on rigorous scientific evidence supplemented by the 'grey literature' where necessary. A lengthy process of consultation and refinement led to the final version that was approved by both WHO and UNICEF.

NICE (England and Wales) systematic reviews of child safety interventions

These reviews cover safety primarily on the roads and in the home. They also address home safety equipment and risk assessment schemes, as well as legislation, regulations and standards for an economic perspective and the effectiveness of strategies. The reviewers adopted a rigorous methodology based entirely on research quality criteria and emphasised that their analyses have both strengths and limitations that readers should consider:

❑ *Home safety equipment installation and risk assessments*: For both of these interventions, the NICE reviewers reported disappointing results. Many of the published studies evaluated impact by means of proxy measures such as the use of safety equipment rather than injury rates. One study (Watson *et al.*, 2005) actually reported an increase injury rates in the intervention group following home safety audits, possibly due to the participants feeling more confident about presenting to emergency departments without being judged adversely. Overall, the evidence for both interventions, separately or in combinations, seems to be weak.

❑ *Cost-effectiveness of legislation, regulation and standards*: Only four interventions of this type survived intensive critical scrutiny: the compulsory wearing of bicycle helmets, the mandatory installation of domestic hot water thermostatic mixing valves, the mandatory installation of smoke detectors in homes, and the use of cameras to enforce speed limits.

❑ *Road safety*: Only 20 mph zones appeared strongly evidence-based measures in terms of reduction in injury incidence. Area-wide traffic-calming interventions, although not achieving statistical significance, were reported to produce injury reductions so consistently that the reviewers felt these studies to be 'indicative of a positive effect'.

❑ *Safety strategies*: The report on safety strategies was more comprehensive in nature than the others and addresses the child safety challenge as a whole. It takes account of the evidence base, cost-effectiveness (where available) and expert opinion. The (provisional) recommendations were detailed and far-reaching and are reproduced below in outline form (NICE, 2010).

NICE advised the UK government as follows:

❑ The government should set targets, in all White Papers and policy plans relevant to child health, for the reduction in child injury incidence.

❑ Action should be cross-governmental and highlight social inequalities in risk.

❑ Local child injury prevention coordinators should be appointed (by the local authority, National Health Service or other agency, or by a joint appointment) to raise awareness of the topic, offer information and advice, help to develop injury prevention strategies within local plans and monitor progress.

❑ Multiple emergency department attendances for injury should be identified by emergency department staff and others and followed up by liaison health visitors.

❑ Training courses, modules and standards should be developed for public health specialists, local injury prevention coordinators and the wider childcare workforce to build capacity.

❑ A national resource for injury surveillance, comprising a network of agencies coordinated by a central point, should be established. As part of surveillance, a robust national emergency department minimum dataset should be created with an enhanced data set operated by a representative sample of hospitals. Data should be shared across agencies, disseminated locally and regionally and subjected to quality control.

❑ Home safety assessments, linked where appropriate to equipment installation schemes, should be performed routinely in all families with a child under 5 within the Healthy Child Programme, taking account of circumstances (including cultural and religious beliefs, and whether residents have the power to implement safety measures). The equipment to be installed in all social and rented housing comprises hard-wired or long-life battery-operated smoke detectors, thermostatic mixing valves for baths, window restrictors and carbon monoxide detectors.

- ❏ Water safety information and skill development should be undertaken in schools and leisure settings.
- ❏ Cycle helmet wearing should be promoted by retailers, schools and cycling event organisers, and campaigns should be evaluated.
- ❏ The national firework safety campaign should be continued and monitored. (The Child Accident Prevention Trust, Royal Society for the Prevention of Accidents [RoSPA] and other agencies offer simple tips for firework safety – see Box 6.1).
- ❏ Play policies should be developed that allow all children to participate in a variety of play and leisure activities. Playgrounds, fairgrounds, swimming pools and toys should comply with British and European safety standards.
- ❏ Local highway authorities should conduct local road safety reviews, including consultations with children, every 2 years. Local road safety partnerships, involving the police, highway agencies and health staff, should be established. Road safety initiatives, using educational, enforcement and engineering measures, should be promoted.

NICE commented on the relative paucity of high-quality research on which to base many of their recommendations. Many of the recommendations are generic, emphasising overarching principles such as the need for intersectoral collaboration, social inclusion, sensitivity to local needs and preferences, and an awareness of child development.

Box 6.1 The RoSPA Firework Code
(www.saferfireworks.com/firework_code/index.htm accessed 7 February 2011)

Ten firework safety tips for adults

Young people should watch and enjoy fireworks at a safe distance and follow the safety rules for using sparklers. Only adults should deal with firework displays and the lighting of fireworks. They should also take care of the safe disposal of fireworks once they have been used.

1 Plan your firework display to make it safe and enjoyable.

2 Keep fireworks in a closed box and use them one at a time.

3 Read and follow the instructions on each firework using a torch if necessary.

4 Light the firework at arm's length with a taper and stand well back.

5 Keep naked flames, including cigarettes, away from fireworks.

6 Never return to a firework once it has been lit.

7 Don't put fireworks in pockets and never throw them.

8 Direct any rocket fireworks well away from spectators.

9 Never use paraffin or petrol on a bonfire.

10 Make sure that the fire is out and surroundings are made safe before leaving.

Taking the various available sources of evidence together, the top-priority recommendations – as adjudged and selected by the author – for unintentional child injury prevention are summarised below. They are neither comprehensive nor immutable and should be continuously reviewed in the light of emerging evidence and interpretation. They describe, in outline, those interventions that have been shown to reduce injury incidence, severity or risk. Some researchers and practitioners have argued that risk reduction is a valuable intermediate indicator when it is not possible or feasible to use injury incidence as an outcome. (Where interventions have been shown to reduce injury risk rather than incidence or severity, their status is inevitably somewhat contentious.)

What works in unintentional child injury prevention? A synthesis

The measures are presented under four headings:

11. Interventions that reduce injury incidence, severity or risk – roads.
12. Interventions that reduce injury incidence, severity or risk – homes.
13. Interventions that reduce injury incidence, severity or risk – elsewhere.
14. Infrastructure interventions that promote safety.

Interventions that reduce injury incidence, severity or risk – roads:

- ❏ Apply area-wide urban safety measures.
- ❏ Promote average traffic speed reduction in both residential and rural areas.
- ❏ Improve enforcement of seat belt/child restraint legislation.
- ❏ Encourage universal bicycle/motorcycle helmet wearing.
- ❏ Facilitate modifications to vehicle design.
- ❏ Implement community-based education/advocacy measures to protect pedestrians.

Interventions that reduce injury incidence, severity or risk – homes:

- ❏ Promote the use of child-resistant closures and packaging.
- ❏ Provide, distribute, install and maintain smoke detectors/alarms/sprinklers
- ❏ Ensure a safe temperature of domestic hot water via thermostatic mixing valves.
- ❏ Install window safety mechanisms to prevent falls from heights.
- ❏ Encourage the installation of stair gates at the tops of stairs.
- ❏ Implement parenting support/early intervention home visiting programmes.
- ❏ Seek to eliminate or modify baby walkers.
- ❏ Seek to eliminate or modify cigarette lighters and cigarettes (self-extinguishing).
- ❏ Promote the sale and wearing of non-flammable sleepwear.

Interventions that reduce injury incidence, severity or risk – elsewhere:

- ❑ Promote the use of personal flotation devices for water recreation.
- ❑ Increase the presence of adequately trained lifeguards at water recreational facilities.
- ❑ Seek the implementation of isolation fencing around private swimming pools.
- ❑ Construct energy-absorbent surfaces in playgrounds.
- ❑ Install playground equipment of an appropriate height (1.5 m for young children)

Infrastructure interventions that promote safety:

- ❑ Develop comprehensive population-wide safety strategies and implementation plans.
- ❑ Identify strong leadership for developing vision, direction and integration.
- ❑ Improve national, regional and local injury data collection, dissemination and use.
- ❑ Create a focal point to plan, implement and evaluate safety measures.
- ❑ Enhance the capacity and infrastructure for injury prevention.
- ❑ Allocate resources for undertaking research, development, monitoring and evaluation.

Each of these measures will now be considered in turn.

Interventions that reduce injury incidence, severity or risk – roads

Apply area-wide urban safety measures

The notion of an 'accident black spot' on our roads is extremely pervasive. It derives from the premise that the roads are basically safe except for defined locations that are hazardous to road users. Although there is some truth in this idea, it is also highly misleading. Some road casualties appear to cluster at specific places but many – probably most – do not. A study of the geography of pedestrian injuries in Montreal (Morency and Cloutier 2006) reported that so-called 'blacks spots' (where there had been at least eight pedestrian victims over 5 years) represented only 1% of intersections where there had been at least one victim. By contrast, in some central boroughs, motorists injured pedestrians in a quarter of all intersections, suggesting that comprehensive, area-wide countermeasures rather than highly targeted ones were necessary.

◄ LEARNING POINT ──────────────────────────

The notion of an 'accident black spot' is misleading. Some road casualties appear to cluster at specific places but many – probably most – do not.
• •

The WHO endorses the area-wide strategy and advocates a 'systems' approach whereby the needs of children are addressed through the design and management of the whole road system rather than focusing on children's behaviour or on highly localised parts of the road system. Altering the physical and traffic flow characteristics of an entire geographical area in a way that reduces the risk of road casualties is a form of primary prevention or, in Haddon Matrix terms, an intervention in the pre-injury phase.

Area-wide measures are those that are designed to reduce risk to pedestrians and other road users throughout a neighbourhood or community rather than at specific locations. They include the introduction and enforcement of speed limits, the creation of safe play areas away from traffic, creating safe routes for children to get to and from school, better illumination of roads at night, engineering measures that separate pedestrians from vehicles or cyclists from vehicles, traffic speed reduction through area-wide engineering and design features of carriageways, and the implementation of awareness-raising safety campaigns. In this way, the level of exposure to risk is reduced for the whole population of the area rather than just the small number who use specific junctions or other locations. Inevitably, there is s a degree of overlap between an area-wide, systems approach and other more targeted strategies.

◄ PRACTICE NUGGET ► ──────────────────────────────

Area-wide urban safety measures include:
- ■ the introduction and enforcement of speed limits;
- ■ the creation of safe play areas away from traffic;
- ■ creating safe routes for children to get to and from school;
- ■ better illumination of roads at night;
- ■ engineering measures that separate pedestrians from vehicles or cyclists from vehicles;
- ■ traffic speed reduction through engineering and design features;
- ■ the implementation of awareness-raising safety campaigns.

───

Promote average traffic speed reduction in both residential and rural areas
Traffic speed is a key causal factor in road traffic injuries, and average traffic speed is generally closely correlated with crash risk. Or, to put it another way, speed is a causal factor in a substantial proportion (around a third) of serious road casualties. Pedestrians and cyclists have much higher survival rates at collision speeds of below 30 km/h (Peden *et al.*, 2004). Speeding (i.e. knowingly exceeding posted speed limits) by drivers is so widespread that it is virtually regarded as the norm, even by police enforcers, in most countries. Speed control is a thus a specialised form of risk reduction. Both Sweden (Vision Zero) and The Netherlands (Sustainable Safety) have made a major commitment to reducing traffic speed in their countries, with impressive results.

■LEARNING POINT────────────────────

Traffic speed is a key causal factor in road safety. It is present in a substantial proportion (around a third) of serious road casualties. The introduction of 20 mph (32 km/h) limits in some urban areas of the UK has resulted in a marked reduction in child pedestrian fatalities.
● ●

Speed reduction interventions have already been mentioned in relation to area-wide measures but are important enough to highlight separately here. They include traffic calming through infrastructural engineering measures (speed humps, mini-roundabouts, pedestrian islands, designated pedestrian crossings and traffic redistribution) prominent speed limit signs with 30 km/h as the norm in residential areas or near schools), raising driver awareness through mass media campaigns, aggressive policing of speed limits, and speed cameras.

■PRACTICE NUGGET────────────────────

Traffic speed reduction interventions include:
- ■ traffic calming through infrastructural engineering measures (speed humps, mini-roundabouts, pedestrian islands, designated pedestrian crossings and traffic redistribution);
- ■ prominent speed limit signs with 30 km/h as the norm in residential areas or near schools;
- ■ raising driver awareness through mass media campaigns;
- ■ aggressive policing of speed limits;
- ■ speed cameras.

The installation of speed cameras at alleged black spots may well be followed by a reduction in crash rates at the camera site. Yet the population as a whole may not experience a statistically significant reduction in casualty rates as most crashes may occur away from camera sites, the selection of the sites may be flawed, the casualty rates at the sites would have declined anyway (regression to the mean) or the crashes have been displaced elsewhere.

The driving public, incited by elements of the mass media, is often resistant or even hostile to traffic-calming measures. Speed cameras are regarded as an unnecessary and ineffective curtailment of 'normal' driving practices and are sometimes regarded as a subterfuge for generating income for either local or national government. These views may be misguided but are firmly held and have a political impact to which politicians feel obliged to respond. Engineering measures, such as speed humps, are denounced as potential lethal hazards to vehicles rather than as a form of road safety. Countering such ill-informed or malicious views is a major challenge that may prove difficult or impossible. Nevertheless, there is undoubtedly a major role for vigorous and effective public information, awareness-raising and education to support valuable environmental and legislative measures.

A combination of all three types of measure – engineering, enforcement and education – may be more effective. The introduction of 20 mph (32 km/h) limits in urban areas of the UK such as parts of London (Grundy *et al.*, 2009) has resulted in a marked reduction in child pedestrian fatalities.

Rural roads are particularly hazardous for a variety of reasons – average speeds are higher, carriageways may be narrower, lighting may be poor. Moreover, some road users may complacently believe that they are at lower risk because of the absence of heavy traffic and relative lack of police enforcement. Paradoxically, low traffic densities remove an important barrier to crashes – slow-moving traffic. The net result of all of this is that crashes tend to occur at higher speeds in environmentally adverse conditions. The severity of injuries is often higher and the availability of emergency services, including a hospital emergency department or trauma centre, much lower than in urban areas.

Improve enforcement of seat belt/child restraint legislation

Although seat belts were invented in the early part of the 20th century, they were not routinely fitted to vehicles until long after that. The legal requirement for drivers and passengers to wear a seat belt was not introduced until much later partly due to a combination of public resistance and political vacillation. Most of that initial opposition and scepticism has disappeared, but compliance rates remain highly variable. Most experts now agree that seat belts have saved countless lives since they were introduced on a wide scale in the 1970s. Large numbers of fatal or life-threatening head injuries and disfiguring facial lacerations are prevented or minimised by reducing the likelihood of car occupants colliding with the windscreen or being thrown from the vehicle in a crash. There is little doubt that total compliance with legislation would further reduce injury incidence and severity.

◾ LEARNING POINT

Seat belts have saved countless lives since they were introduced. They have particularly prevented life-threatening head injuries and disfiguring facial lacerations.

In the case of young children (under about 10 years of age), the wearing of seat belts is a more complex matter owing to the need to take account of their very different physiognomies from those of adults. For decades, seat belts were designed exclusively for adults and large numbers of unrestrained children were killed or injured in car crashes. Nowadays, under pressure from governments, consumers and legislation, manufacturers have responded to this need by producing a range of restraints and booster seats.

Child restraints in vehicles are of three types:

❑ rear-facing restraints for infants;
❑ forward-facing restraints;
❑ booster cushions or seats for older children.

These restraints are highly effective – they reduce the risk of death or serious injuries in crashes by at least 50% (Peden *et al.*, 2008). Yet, even in countries with strict legislation, compliance is often poor or children are restrained in inappropriate devices. Measures that appear to increase the use of child restraints include legislation backed by enforcement, publicity campaigns and the free or reduced-cost distribution of restraints to families.

In 2006, the UK law changed to require all children aged under 3 years to be restrained in an appropriate child seat. The new rules are fairly complex and are explained by the Automobile Association as shown in Box 6.2 and summarised in the table in the box.

Box 6.2 UK rules for child restraints in vehicles

(www.theaa.com/motoring_advice/child_safety/seatbelts.html accessed 7 February 2011)

The rules – since September 2006

All children under three years old *must use an appropriate child restraint* when travelling in any car or goods vehicle (except in the rear of a taxi if a child seat is not available). Children aged three or more years old and up to 135cm (approx 4ft 5in) in height *must use an appropriate child restraint* when travelling in cars or goods vehicles fitted with seat belts. (Few exceptions are permitted.) Rear-facing baby seats must not be used in seats with an active frontal air-bag.

The number of people carried in the rear of vehicles may not exceed the number of seats available fitted with seat belts or child restraints. Only child restraints complying with UN ECE Reg 44.03 or a later standard may be used. In a vehicle without seat belts (e.g. a classic car), children 3 years and over can only travel in the back, and those under 3 years cannot be carried at all.

Drivers remain responsible for seat belt wearing and use of the relevant child seat or booster by children under 14 years of age. There is a special exemption for children over 3 years on an occasional journey (e.g. unforeseen emergency) over a short distance. The child must still use an adult belt and sit in the rear. This exemption is not for journeys such as the regular school run.

PRACTICE NUGGET

The **key seat belt/child restraint rules** in the UK are as follows:

- Children under 3 years of age must always have a child seat – except when they travel in the rear of taxis and a child seat is not available.

- Children aged 3 or more years old and up to 135 cm (approx 4 ft 5 in) in height must use an appropriate child restraint when travelling in cars or goods vehicles fitted with seat belts.

- Rear-facing baby seats must not be used in seats with an frontal air-bag.

- The number of people carried in the rear of vehicles may not exceed the number of seats available fitted with seat belts or child restraints.

- Drivers remain responsible for seat belt wearing and use of the relevant child seat or booster by children under 14 years of age.

Person in car	Front seat	Rear seat
Summary table of UK legislation on vehicle restraints *Source:* Automobile Association 2010		
Driver	A seat belt **must** be worn if fitted.	
Child under 3 years	The correct child seat **must** be used.	The correct child seat **must** be used. If one is not available in a taxi, a child may travel unrestrained.
Child 3 to 11 years and under 135cm (approx 4ft 5in)	The correct child restraint **must** be used.	The correct child restraint must be used where seatbelts are fitted. A child must use an adult belt in the rear if: <ul><li>in a taxi the correct child restraint is not available</li><li>on a short and occasional trip, the child restraint is not available</li><li>two occupied child restraints prevent use of a third</li></ul>
Child 12 or 13 (or younger child over 135cm)	A seat belt **must** be worn if fitted.	A seat belt **must** be worn if fitted.
Adult passenger	A seat belt **must** be worn if fitted.	A seat belt **must** be worn if fitted.

Encourage universal bicycle/motorcycle helmet wearing

Cyclists sustain a range of injuries, but the most serious are undoubtedly those to the head. Although the need to protect children's brains from injury in the course of being carried on a motorcycle is widely accepted (although far from universally implemented), governments have been slow to promote cycle helmet use either through public awareness campaigns or through legislation (three notable exceptions being Australia, Canada and the USA). This resistance is somewhat baffling given the strong evidence from case-control studies that helmets reduce the risk of severe head injury by at least two-thirds (Thompson *et al.*, 2005) and are especially likely to be effective when cyclists are involved in incidents that do not involve a collision with other vehicles (Hynd *et al.*, 2009).

Legislation has been shown to increase helmet wearing to at least 90% (Karkhaneh *et al.*, 2006) with a consequent reduction in serious head injuries to cyclists – 45% in the case of the Canadian provinces. Some sceptics (Robinson, 2006) claim that this is due to reduced exposure owing to fewer children cycling, and that any health gains achieved in this way are likely to be more than offset by the consequent reduction in the level of exercise taken by children.

◖LEARNING POINT▶───────────────────────────────

Legislation has been shown to increase bicycle helmet wearing to at least 90% with a consequent reduction in serious head injuries to cyclists – 45% in the case of the Canadian provinces.
● ●

The Netherlands is an oft-cited example of a country where cycling is common yet head injury is rare. This is a myth. Although the road environment is certainly safer for cyclists in that country than in most other places, Dutch crash data clearly show that cycling is associated with an elevated risk of serious injury. Children aged 4–8 years are most likely to be involved in a crash and suffer brain injury (World Health Organization, 2006). On the other hand, older children are arguably more likely to be exposed to heavy traffic.

There are several obstacles to the universal wearing of helmets that injury prevention practitioners should bear in mind. One is cost, and some form of subsidy may be necessary to enhance their affordability to poorer families. A second is the need to ensure a helmet of appropriate size and design to protect the child. In this respect, the promulgation and enforcement of manufacturing standards is critical. A third is the difficulty of ensuring that the helmet fits the child's growing head comfortably and safely. A fourth is the tendency of some children (especially teenagers) – and some parents – to resist the wearing of helmets on aesthetic grounds. Enabling children to choose their own helmets may be helpful. Finally, parents often try to insist on their children wearing helmets while they themselves do not, a parenting strategy that is doomed to failure.

In the UK, despite the absence of legislation, the Bicycle Helmet Initiative Trust (www.bhit.org/ accessed 7 February 2011) is in no doubt that the balance of research favours cycle helmet wearing, as does the WHO Helmet Initiative (www.whohelmets.org/ accessed 7 February 2011).

◖PRACTICE NUGGET▶───────────────────────────────

When promoting cycle helmet wearing, practitioners should remember that:
- cycle helmets greatly reduce the risk of serious head injury;
- legislation, although rare, is effective in promoting helmet wearing and reducing injuries;
- some form of subsidy may be necessary to enhance their affordability to poorer families;
- a helmet should be of appropriate size, design and manufacturing standard;
- a helmet should fit the child's growing head comfortably and safely;
- children (especially teenagers) should be permitted to choose their own helmets;
- parents should act as role models and wear helmets themselves.

Facilitate modifications to vehicle design

The striking reduction in serious road casualty rates over the past few decades in many countries has been attributed to many factors, one of the most influential of which has been the improvement in the characteristics of vehicles. Engineering and technological advances in vehicle design and manufacture, often backed by regulatory standards, have undoubtedly contributed substantially to safety, although this is hard to quantify. These have taken the form of both primary and secondary preventive measures. Many of these were brought about by the vehicle manufacturing industry itself, albeit under consumer and governmental pressure.

Here are a few examples that have been especially important in protecting children either as passengers or pedestrians:

- ❏ improved braking, lighting, suspension and road-holding features that reduce the incidence of crashes;
- ❏ more effective energy-absorbing crumple zones and side impact bars that reduce the risk of intrusion of another vehicle or object into the passenger compartment;
- ❏ less damaging external surfaces of vehicle fronts that reduce the severity of injuries to pedestrians;
- ❏ internal fixture points for the fitting of restraints (see above);
- ❏ the use of audible alarms and reversing lights to reduce the risk to pedestrians when reversing;
- ❏ the incorporation of alcohol interlock (alcolock) devices to immobilise the ignition if the driver's breath contains alcohol.

There remains considerable scope for improved safety through better vehicle design. Among the measures that would help to achieve this objective are raising public and political awareness of the importance of vehicle characteristics in road safety, passing and enforcing legislation that optimises the roadworthiness and safety of all vehicles, old and new, in all countries of the world (as 90% of fatal crashes occur in low- or middle-income countries that contain only 4% of the world's vehicles), and investing in research that strives to produce further improvements to vehicle safety.

◄PRACTICE NUGGET

Further improvements to road vehicle design may be achieved by:

- ■ raising public and political awareness of the importance of vehicle characteristics in road safety;
- ■ passing and enforcing legislation that optimises the roadworthiness and safety of all vehicles, old and new, in all countries of the world;
- ■ investing in research that strives to produce further improvements to vehicle safety.

Implement community-based education/advocacy measures to protect pedestrians
Generally speaking, educational interventions have shown minimal results in terms of injury incidence. A systematic review (Turner *et al.*, 2004), however, of community-based programmes concluded (on the basis of only four studies) that such programmes, particularly if properly resourced and combined with social and environmental strategies, could achieve reductions of up to about half of pedestrian injuries.

Multifaceted programmes that are focused on child pedestrian skills training, such as Injury Minimization Programme for Schools in England and Kerbcraft in Scotland aimed at primary school children (Thomson and Whelan 1997), have shown positive results on knowledge and behaviour, although impacts on injury incidence have been more difficult to discern (Duperrex *et al.*, 2002). These interventions are more likely to succeed when they have a strong emphasis on the experiential learning of practical skills, when parents are closely involved and when the programmes fit well with local and national educational curricula. Some of these initiatives have a wider remit than pedestrian safety and include, for example, safety education in simulated environments, cycle training and experience, enhanced conspicuousness using highly visible coloured items of clothing or other equipment, and first aid training.

PRACTICE NUGGET

Community- and school-based **educational programmes designed to protect pedestrians** seem more likely to succeed if:
■ learning is experiential rather than didactic;
■ parents are closely involved;
■ teaching is multifaceted and includes road safety in general
■ programmes fit well into local and national curricula.

Advocacy, per se, has a long and illustrious tradition in the injury prevention field. A modern and highly effective pioneer of road safety was Ralph Nader (1965). Since then, many community and parental advocacy groups have been established and have achieved high-profile media coverage that impinges, to varying degrees, on the political landscape. Some of these groups have, however, adopted positions (e.g. opposition to speed cameras) that defy both the available evidence and rationale analysis and may contribute to political pressures to abandon safety measures of established efficacy.

Interventions that reduce injury incidence, severity or risk – homes
Promote the use of child-resistant closures and packaging
Because very young children are particularly exposed to the risks of poisonings and ingestions, preventive strategies have to be directed at either their parents or the

home environment. Medicines, solvents and other household chemicals are often involved. Efforts to render their storage and packaging 'child-proof' have yielded better results than either exhortations or educational measures directed at parents or carers. This is because all young children are naturally curious and will explore their environment by reaching out to an appealing-looking item and placing it in their mouth. Nevertheless, these containers are not child-proof.

◀ LEARNING POINT ────────────────────────

Efforts to render the storage and packaging of medicines and household chemicals 'child-proof' have yielded better results, in terms of poisoning prevention, than educational measures directed at parents or carers.
· ·

The strongest risk factor for the ingestion of a harmful product by a child is its accessibility. Keeping a dangerous product out reach of children is the most important countermeasure, followed by ensuring that the contents of a container are inaccessible to a child. Striking and sustained reductions in unintentional poisoning rates and fatalities have been demonstrated in England and Wales (Flanagan *et al.*, 2005) and the USA (Walton, 1982) following the introduction of child-resistant packaging or storage, usually mandated by legislation. The European Union has, since 1998, required the storage of toxic substances in child-resistant containers that are clearly and appropriately labelled, in places that are not within reach of children or near to foodstuffs, and labelled in such a way that the substances in question cannot be mistaken for food. Initial costs to manufacturers and distributors are, over time, greatly outweighed by the savings accruing from avoiding the treatment costs of poisonings.

There is some controversy around blister packs (or non-reclosable packaging), a form of child-resistant packaging that is growing in popularity, as they may merely delay or limit access by a child to a tablet or capsule. Nevertheless, they do appear to be effective in reducing the risk of poisoning through the unintentional ingestion by children of potentially dangerous medication such as paracetamol (Turvill *et al.*, 2000). Other measures taken recently that have reduced mortality and morbidity from poisoning include limiting the number of tablets or capsules per dose prescribed or sold over the counter in a bottle, and improved acute medical care.

Despite the best efforts of all concerned, and practical preventive advice that is freely disseminated by the UK Child Accident Prevention Trust (www.capt.org.uk/resources/talking-about-poisons accessed 25 February 2011) and other organisations, children will occasionally ingest a potentially harmful substance. Local poison control centres are potentially helpful sources of advice for parents and carers, although they may be relatively inaccessible to the general public.

━PRACTICE NUGGET━━━━━━━━━━━━━━━━━━━━━━━━━━━━

To prevent poisonings in the home, the **Child Accident Prevention Trust** stresses these points:

■ Household chemicals and medicines should be stored out of the sight and reach of young children, preferably in a locked cupboard. Garden or DIY products should also be locked away. Don't store medicines in the fridge.

■ All medicines or household chemicals should be kept in their original containers as this helps both children and adults recognise dangerous substances.

■ Child-resistant containers are not child-proof, and many 4- or 5-year-olds can undo these tops. Child-resistant caps work by slowing down rather than preventing a child's access to dangerous substances.

■ Some household chemicals are sold with a bittering agent in them so that if children do get the substance in their mouth, they are likely to spit it out immediately.

Provide, distribute, install and maintain smoke detectors/alarms/sprinklers
While burns and scalds are the most numerous fire- or heat-related injuries to children in the home, the most frequent cause of death is lung damage due to smoke inhalation. It is also perhaps the most amenable to prevention of all fire-related injuries.

━LEARNING POINT━━━━━━━━━━━━━━━━━━━━━━━━━━━━

While burns and scalds are the most numerous fire- or heat-related injuries to children in the home, the most frequent cause of death is smoke inhalation. The fitting of smoke detectors is a form of secondary prevention that has been shown to reduce the risk of death by almost three-quarters.
● ●

The fitting of smoke detectors is a form of secondary prevention (operating at the 'event' phase of the Haddon Matrix) that has been shown to reduce the risk of death in house fires by almost three-quarters (Runyan *et al.*, 1992). This simple technological advance was initially hampered by two main factors: batteries that ran down or were removed, and cost. Both have been overcome in recent years by hard-wiring of the alarms to the household electrical supply, and mass production respectively. More recently still, a further technological breakthrough has been achieved by linking the alarms to water sprinklers, although these have so far been taken up by commercial organisations to a greater extent than by the residential sector. Sprinklers are now so sophisticated that they will quickly douse a fire in a highly localised space rather than cause generalised flooding of the property.

Systematic reviews of randomised controlled trials have suggested that education alone produces minimal benefit while distribution combined with installation makes a greater impact. The most effective strategy, however, is a combination of education, installation and legislation (Ballasteros *et al.*, 2005). Because house fires are strongly socially patterned, targeting of smoke detector installation and upkeep is especially worthwhile in poorer areas (Mallonee, 2000). Given that all households are at potential risk, however, and that targeting is not always a panacea and may be complicated to administer, the universal protection of all residential properties, starting with the older housing stock, seems the most sensible policy. Moreover, smoke detectors represent a staggeringly good investment, saving nearly $30 for every $1 spent (Miller and Hendrie, 2005).

Fire safety training, especially when experiential methods are used, has been shown to improve the knowledge and behaviour of both children and parents, although reductions in injury or fire incidence have not been demonstrated.

▬◖PRACTICE NUGGET ◗▬▬▬▬▬▬▬▬▬▬

Smoke alarms may be effective in reducing house fire casualties if:

■ a combination of education, installation and legislation is used;

■ poorer areas are prioritised in the context of universal provision;

■ initial costs are offset against future returns;

■ other fire prevention measures, such as fire guards and the safe storage of matches and candles, are also taken.

Ensure a safe temperature of domestic hot water via thermostatic mixing valves
Scalds are among the most frequently occurring and distressing injuries in young children. They are due to the spillage of boiling or even moderately hot liquids onto the vulnerable and easily damaged skin on exposed surfaces. The sources are mainly drinks, kettles or pans and baths.

Because prognosis, in terms of survival and morbidity, is correlated with the percentage of the total body surface that is damaged, bath water scalds to infants and young children tend to be the most serious, causing long periods of hospitalisation, prolonged pain, scarring and disability, and very high healthcare costs. Sensible strategies to prevent bath water scalding include pouring cold water into a bath before adding hot water, and providing constant supervision of young children at bath time. A highly effective means of risk reduction is to fit thermostatic mixing valves to hot water taps in domestic bathrooms. In this way, maximum temperatures of 50°C or less can be achieved, with consequent reductions in scald incidence and severity. (Lower temperatures are usually considered undesirable, in terms of both the risk of *Legionella* infection and acceptability to householders.)

Studies from the USA (Feldman, 1998; Rivara, 1998), Canada (Han *et al.*, 2007) and elsewhere have confirmed that a combination of legislation and education with regard to scald risk can reap great benefits. Australia, for example, is one of the first countries to mandate a maximum temperature of 50°C for hot water taps in bathrooms, for both new installations and replacements.

◀LEARNING POINT▶━━━━━━━━━━━━━━━━━━━━━━━━━━━━━━

A highly effective means of scald risk reduction is to fit thermostatic mixing valves to hot water taps in domestic bathrooms. Maximum temperatures of 50°C or less can be achieved with consequent reductions in scald incidence and severity.
• •

◀PRACTICE NUGGET▶━━━━━━━━━━━━━━━━━━━━━━━━━━━

Sensible **bath scald prevention strategies** include:
■ pouring cold water into a bath before adding hot water;

■ providing constant supervision of young children at bath time;

■ fitting thermostatic mixing valves to domestic bath taps to maintain hot tap temperatures at lower than 50°C;

■ combining education with legislation on fitting thermostatic mixing valves

Install window safety mechanisms to prevent falls from heights
Falls are common in childhood and are a normal part of development. Minor injuries (lacerations, bruises and minor fractures) caused by falls frequently present to emergency departments; many of these are hard to avoid and, perhaps, not worthy of attention. In a minority of cases, falls can cause severe, disabling or even fatal injury. These injuries, affecting mainly the limbs and the skull, not only cause much suffering, but are also costly to healthcare systems and the wider society.

Falls from the windows of high buildings are associated with high rates of death and disability in children. Although encouraging parental supervision of young children is always logical and mostly helpful, modifying the environment – such as by fitting window bars and locks – tends to yield greater public health returns. A study in the 1970s from a low-income area of New York, called the Children Can't Fly programme (Spiegel and Lindaman, 1977), from the City Department of Health, demonstrated a reduction of 50% in 2 years of reported falls from high-rise buildings following implementation of three components. These were a systematic, voluntary reporting system, a parental education service allied with a mass media campaign, and the free distribution of easily installable window guards to families with pre-school-age children. Impressed by the initial results, the New York Department of Health mandated that, by 1979, all owners of multiple dwellings in the city had to provide window guards in homes where children aged under 11 resided. There is little doubt that the passage and enforcement of building regulations to ensure that such guards are fitted as a matter of course generates even greater benefits than intermittent campaigns or programmes.

The UK Child Accident Prevention Trust (www.capt.org.uk/) offers several specific pieces of advice to parents and carers intent on preventing young children suffering serious falls: to keep furniture such as beds and chairs away from windows, to fit window locks or safety catches to stop windows opening more than 6.5 cm (2.5

inches), and to ensure that family members know where keys are kept in case of fire. They add that research indicates that parents are more concerned about fire safety and think that window locks will hamper their evacuation. An additional message is needed – that the keys need to be kept close by.

◄ PRACTICE NUGGET ►

To prevent young children suffering serious falls in the home:
- keep furniture such as beds and chairs away from windows;
- fit window locks or safety catches to stop windows opening more than 6.5 cm (2.5 inches);
- ensure that family members know where keys are kept in case of fire.

Encourage the installation of stair gates at the tops of stairs
Falling down a staircase can cause serious injury to a child, because of both the heights involved and the risk of striking physical protuberances or hard surfaces on the way down. Poor lighting, cluttered floors, frayed carpets and a generally poor-quality physical environment increase the likelihood of severe injury. Upper limb injuries are particularly common in children aged over 1 year as they will try to protect themselves using their arms.

Stair gates fitted at the tops of stairs (and sometimes at the foot) are believed to reduce the risk of fall injuries in young, mobile children. There are two basic types: screw fitting and pressure fitting. The former requires secure fitting to a wall or stairwell frame, and may need the help of a tradesman. The latter type is easier to install but should not be used at the top of a staircase. Some gates close automatically, whereas others do not.

◄ PRACTICE NUGGET ►

To **prevent staircase falls** in the home:
- keep floors well lit and clear of toys and other clutter;
- fit stair gates (of the appropriate standard) at the top and bottom of the stairs;
- ensure that parents know how to fit stair gates securely;
- encourage parents to teach children how to use stairs safely;
- emphasise the importance of continuous supervision of young children.

As with all safety devices, the setting of a standard by national or international statutory authorities can be a useful means of ensuring consistency of protection and of reassuring parents. There is a British Safety Standard (EN 1930) for stair gates designed to protect children under 24 months, although RoSPA has raised some concerns about the extent to which the standard is met by products on the UK market in the early 2000s (www.rospa.com/HomeSafety/Info/stairgates-en1930.

pdf accessed 7 February 2011). The correct use of such devices cannot, of course, be assumed. Home safety educational campaigns have shown modest impacts on parental awareness, the appropriate use of stair gates and, occasionally, small reductions in fall rates (Kendrick *et al.*, 2009).

Implement parenting support/early intervention home visiting programmes

The growing recognition of the crucial importance of a child's early experience in determining a range of outcomes has major implications for injury prevention. This operates both directly and indirectly. First, parents and carers are the 'front-line personnel' who provide immediate physical protection for children. If that protection is inadequate or withdrawn, through either neglect or abuse, children are liable to suffer injuries. Second, a warm, nurturing and empathetic emotional environment is essential for normal child development, mental and physical health and educational achievement. Its absence will adversely impact on the child throughout life, and one manifestation of this is a higher risk of injury.

Parenting programmes that involve home visiting and intensive interaction with parents, such as Incredible Years (Barlow, 2007), the Nurse–Family Partnership (Olds and Henderson, 1986) and Triple P (Sanders, 2008), have shown positive results in terms of child behaviour, development, general health and educational achievement (Geddes *et al.*, 2010). Evidence is accruing that parenting and early intervention programmes (such as the Nurse–Family Partnership, Triple P and Parents as Teachers) increase the uptake and use of domestic safety equipment and reduce the incidence of injuries, both unintentional and intentional (Kendrick *et al.*, 2007; Prinz *et al.*, 2009).

◀ LEARNING POINT ──────────────────────────────

Evidence has begun to accrue that parenting and early intervention programmes can increase the uptake and use of domestic safety equipment and also reduce the incidence of injuries, both unintentional and intentional.
• •

Pathways to greater home safety for children may be either direct, through the identification and removal of physical hazards, or indirect, through improved general parenting skills, or through a combination of the two. Home visits that are explicitly focused on safety (home safety checks) do appear to be effective in reducing risk and promoting safety awareness, although the impact on injury incidence may be less striking (Kendrick *et al.*, 2007). Such visits (performed mainly by health visitors or public health nurses) seem more effective when targeted at high-risk families, when they are age-appropriate and when they are combined with the free or subsidised distribution of safety equipment, although that finding may simply reflect the type of research that has been performed.

█ PRACTICE NUGGET ─────────────────────────────────

Parenting support and home visiting programmes can improve home safety:

■ directly, through the identification and removal of physical hazards via home visits (mainly by public health nurses);

■ indirectly, through improved general parenting skills in the crucial early years of child development .

───

Seek to eliminate or modify baby walkers

Several consumer products used to transport or entertain infants have been shown to be responsible for both fatal and non-fatal injuries. One of these is the infant or baby walker. Parents may be under the mistaken impression that these devices are helpful in exercising their babies or enhance early walking ability. In fact, the opposite may well be true in that they probably actually impair physical and mental development (Petridou *et al.*, 1996). Moreover, walkers expose their occupants to hazards by enabling them to gain access sharp objects and dangerous substances as well as staircases, oven doors and fireplaces, and by tipping the child out of the walker in unexpected locations. These incidents can occur very quickly even when the child is being closely supervised. The most frequent type of walker-related injury is falls, although burns and scalds, lacerations, ingestions and drownings can also occur.

█ LEARNING POINT ───────────────────────────────────

Baby walkers expose their occupants to hazards by enabling them to gain access to sharp objects, dangerous substances, staircases, oven doors and fireplaces, and by tipping the child out of the walker in unexpected locations.
● ●

When these risks became evident in the 1980s and 90s, awareness campaigns and additional labelling were among the strategies employed to try to reduce walker-related injuries, to little effect, although later, more intensive campaigns were more successful (Conners *et al.*, 2002). When the US voluntary standards agency ASTM (formerly the American Society for Testing and Materials, now ASTM International) recommended safer walker designs (and stationary walkers were introduced, such injuries declined steeply but did not disappear. The new European standard requires walkers to move more slowly and stop if a wheel goes over the edge of a step. Some countries, including Canada, have banned the sale, advertising and importation of baby walkers, and that may be the most sensible preventive strategy.

◄ PRACTICE NUGGET ►────────────────────────────────

In addressing the use of baby walkers, remember that:
- many parents have the mistaken belief that they help their child to walk;
- offering advice on walker use is unlikely to make walkers safe;
- stationary devices are probably safer than mobile ones;
- legislation to ban walkers may be the only solution.

Seek to eliminate or modify cigarette lighters and cigarettes (self-extinguishing)

Cigarettes are a threat to more than respiratory health: they also increase the chances of burns, domestic fires, smoke inhalation and death. Cigarette lighters have historically made a significant contribution to this risk. Children are attracted to small, light, shiny objects that spark into flame and will imitate adults by handling them if the opportunity arises. At one time, when smoking prevalence was high and lighters were ubiquitous, scores of children were injured or killed through playing with the product (Smith *et al.*, 1991). The introduction in the USA of a new standard for all lighters produced an immediate and impressive reduction in fires, injuries and deaths, along with enormous financial savings (Smith *et al.*, 2002). A European standard was issued in 2002, and aspects of this were made mandatory by the European Union in 2007. Other parts of the world are likely to follow suit.

The technical ability to manufacture a self-extinguishing or reduced-ignition propensity cigarette (RIP) has existed for several years. The tobacco industry has been reluctant to market such 'fire-safe' products, mainly on cost grounds and also because of a feared backlash from smokers. At the same time, some professionals have been wary of lending support to a so-called 'safer' cigarette in case such an attitude undermines anti-smoking efforts. The net result is that international action has been relatively sluggish despite strong evidence that discarded and still smouldering cigarettes are a major cause of house fires and are responsible for around a third of fire fatalities. Taking the lead from New York State in 2004, most US states now require the industry to conform to an RIP standard, as do Canada and Australia. The European Union is likely to introduce a standard in the near future following intensive lobbying from public health organisations including the European Public Health Alliance (www.epha.org/a/2556 accessed 7 February 2011).

Promote the sale and wearing of non-flamable sleepwear

A productive form of secondary prevention is the passage of consumer product safety standards that reduce the flammability of household materials such as furniture, bed covers and clothing. The need to prohibit the sale of children's nightwear that could easily catch fire causing severe injuries and death was recognised as early as 1813 in England by Newton Bosworth (cited by Jackson, 1995). The textiles used in the manufacture of children's nightwear, such as polyester/cotton blended fibres, were especially prone to ignition from a small flame source such as a lighter or match. The loose-fitting, flowing nature of the clothes, especially those worn by girls, produced a lethal 'chimney effect' that enabled the flame to spread rapidly throughout the garment. The injuries caused in such circumstances are likely to be particularly severe, with consequently high fatality and disability rates, compounded by serious physical and mental scarring of survivors.

◖LEARNING POINT

A productive form of secondary prevention is the passage of consumer product safety standards that reduce the flammability of household materials such as furniture, bed covers and clothing.

Since the latter half of the 20th century, many countries and jurisdictions have passed regulations requiring children's nightwear to be flame-proof. The 1985 UK regulations cover all nightwear including pyjamas and dressing gowns, and require these products to carry a label indicating adherence to a specified standard. Standards vary enormously between countries, and some of the earlier, more stringent regulations have been relaxed amid great controversy. Evaluation studies have generally suggested that these regulations have resulted in a rapid decline in injuries involving nightwear (McLoughlin *et al.*, 1977), although some recent analyses have been more circumspect and have called for tighter regulation (Horrocks *et al.*, 2004).

Three particular problems have arisen in relation to flame-resistant nightwear. First, both manufacturers and consumers have been reluctant to endorse the spraying of nightwear with flame-retardant chemicals as some of these have been suspected of being carcinogenic. Second, there has been an increasing trend in recent years for children to wear T-shirts or other day wear at night, thereby failing to be protected by the regulations. And third, the data available for analysis of the impact of regulation are sparse and frequently inconclusive.

Interventions that reduce injury incidence, severity or risk – elsewhere
Promote the use of personal flotation devices for water recreation

Drowning is usually one of the top three or four causes of child injury deaths around the world. All ages of child are at risk. A small child can drown in just 5 cm of water, shallower than the level in an average paddling pool. Older children, even if they are strong swimmers, can get swept away in the sea by unexpected currents or high waves. US Coast Guard statistics (United States Coast Guard, 2010) demonstrate that the vast majority of drowned victims of boating incidents were not wearing life jackets, although other factors, including weather, alcohol, swimming skill and location, are often involved.

Apart from being exposed to intermittent natural catastrophes such as floods, children are at risk of drowning in domestic baths, garden ponds, open water and swimming pools. These risks are age-related. Many children drown in recreational settings such as on a boat, at the seaside or in a swimming pool or lake. Even if a child can swim, parental or lifeguard supervision is critical in such circumstances but may not always be possible. If a child falls into water, the wearing of a life jacket or other personal flotation device (PFD; a smaller, lighter, more comfortable but less buoyant version of a life jacket) can be life-saving.

◀LEARNING POINT▶

As children may drown in a recreational setting such as on a boat, at the seaside or in a swimming pool or lake, the wearing of a life jacket or other personal flotation device can be life-saving.

PFDs have been designed for use in a range of recreational settings – boating, fishing, water skiing, canoeing, kayaking and rafting. Not all are suitable for small children. As well as buoyancy, size is critical. The PFD should fit snugly but not obstruct breathing. Bright colours are not merely attractive, they also aid visibility in the water. Ideally, the devices should turn the child face upwards, with the head supported and the mouth out of the water. Many countries now require all recreational vessels to carry sufficient numbers of life jackets for all passengers, but these are of much less value if they are not worn at all times. Educational campaigns to increase the wearing of these devices have had some effect, but regulation, backed by enforcement, seems to be the most effective approach (Cassell *et al.*, 2007).

Educating children, parents, carers and others who find themselves responsible for child welfare seems a sensible measure. Water safety should be an essential part of every child's education, including swimming lessons from the age of about 5 years.

◀PRACTICE NUGGET▶

In **promoting PFDs**, remember that:
- the PFD should fit snugly and not obstruct breathing;
- bright colours are not merely attractive, they also aid visibility in water;
- the device should turn the child face upwards, with the head supported and the mouth out of the water;
- the device is of much less value if not worn at all times;
- educational campaigns to increase the wearing of these devices have some effect;
- regulation, backed by enforcement, seems to be the most effective approach.

Increase the presence of adequately trained lifeguards at water recreational facilities
The dangers of water recreation have already been alluded to. Drowning is most

common in children under 5 years of age, particularly in the home. Young children should never be left unsupervised or with another young child in or near even shallow water. Parents tend to overestimate their child's skill in the water. Lifeguards (sometimes known as lifesavers), either voluntary or professional, are an increasingly common sight at beaches and swimming pools around the world despite the paucity of formal evaluation studies of lifeguarding. Two Australian studies (Manolios and Mackie, 1988; Fenner *et al.*, 1995) have, however, offered some encouraging evidence of its effectiveness.

If properly trained and skill levels maintained through supervision and repeated updating (World Health Organization, 2003), lifeguards can contribute to water safety in numerous ways. Their very presence will deter high-risk behaviour. They can act as models of safe behaviour, control the risk-taking actions of swimmers, continuously monitor water and weather conditions, and restrict or prohibit swimming if conditions become too hazardous. They can also intervene after an incident by rescuing swimmers in difficulty or resuscitating swimmers who have inhaled water.

Seek the implementation of isolation fencing around private swimming pools

Children usually love to play in water and should be encouraged to do so. Although all children should learn to swim from an early age (around 5 years), creating a physical barrier between children and a source of danger is a valuable form of passive intervention. Erecting safety barriers or fencing, particularly on all four sides, around pools or spas, both public and private, has been shown to reduce the risk of young children drowning by preventing their access to water (Thompson and Rivara, 2000). Fencing should be secure and have child-proof self-latching gates. In the near future, it may prove possible to create such a barrier through the use of alarm signalling systems rather than a physical structure.

As with many other forms of injury prevention, education or exhortation is insufficient. Awareness-raising campaigns through the mass media or community groups have a place, but optimum results are achieved by the passage of regulations backed by enforcement. All Australian states have pool fence laws, as do several American states, but Europe has been slow to legislate. France, a country with many swimming pools and one of the highest infant drowning rates in the world, passed a law in 2003 requiring most pools to incorporate an approved safety system.

◄ LEARNING POINT ─────────────────────────

Erecting safety barriers or fencing, particularly on all four sides, around pools or spas has been shown to reduce the risk of young children drowning by preventing their access to water.

● ●

━ PRACTICE NUGGET ━━━━━━━━━━━━━━━━━━━━━━━━━━━━━━

To prevent drownings at swimming pools, remember that:

■ all children should learn to swim from about 5 years of age;

■ fencing should be secure and have child-proof, self-latching gates;

■ awareness-raising campaigns through the mass media or community groups have a place but are insufficient;

■ the best results are achieved by the passage of regulations backed by enforcement.

Construct energy-absorbent surfaces in playgrounds

Play, both formal and informal, is an essential part of childhood and normal child development across the physical, social, intellectual and emotional dimensions. Encouraging children to take more exercise is a core objective of obesity prevention strategies and one that can only be realised if parents feel confident that their children can play safely, supervised or not, on equipment that is appropriate for their age, fundamentally safe and adequately maintained. Most neighbourhoods contain one or more playgrounds with equipment of varying quality and levels of maintenance. Until fairly recently, even purpose-built children's playgrounds were constructed of materials such as steel and concrete that virtually guaranteed a high injury rate. Children suffer mainly orthopaedic and head injuries when falling from such equipment and striking either an object or the ground. Some of these injuries may be surprisingly severe and should alert healthcare staff to the possibility of abuse.

Concrete, asphalt or other hard surfaces are unacceptable in modern playgrounds. Grass and packed earth surfaces may become degraded by damp and lose their original physical characteristics. The introduction of energy-absorbent surfaces, such as bark, sand or rubber, has greatly reduced risk (especially of head injury) without impairing activity. The energy-attenuating characteristics of any given surface cannot be assumed on visual inspection. Assessing whether a specified material is of a safe depth and has been subject to adequate maintenance can only be established by expert examination. Playground surfacing standards, with a high level of enforcement, are becoming increasingly popular around the world. Some safety organisations, such as RoSPA in the UK, offer playground inspections to give advice to schools, local authorities and others about playground safety in general and safety standards of equipment and surfaces in particular. Evaluational studies of these standards are rare.

━ LEARNING POINT ━━━━━━━━━━━━━━━━━━━━━━━━━━━━━━

The introduction into children's playgrounds of energy-absorbent surfaces has greatly reduced risk (especially of head injury) without impairing activity.
● ●

None of these design features, however, absolves parents and carers of their responsibility to supervise children carefully at playgrounds. Young children, especially, require close attention and may be too small to use some equipment. All children should be taught how to play safely in playgrounds to minimise the risk of injury to themselves and other children.

◄PRACTICE NUGGET)────────────────────────────

In promoting playground safety, remember that:
- the introduction of playground safety standards has greatly improved playground safety;
- however well designed they are, playgrounds remain unsafe for children in the absence of close adult supervision;
- young children may be too small to use some playgrounds;
- all children should be taught how to play safely in playgrounds.

Install playground equipment of appropriate height (1.5 m for young children)
A second playground structural feature that is relevant to assessing injury risk, and one that is closely interconnected to surface quality, is equipment height. The greater the height, the more likely will a child be injured as a result of falling. High structures, especially if they contain moving or swaying components, are particularly appealing to most children. Children under 5 years of age are at higher risk because they lack sufficient coordination and strength to meet the challenge of a high climbing frame. They also lack the experience or capacity to recognise risk.

Because of the large number of variables (including, for example, the nature of the equipment, the age of the child and whether other children are playing on the structure) involved in determining injury risk, it is far from easy to obtain professional consensus around the determination of maximum height. Studies from Australia (Sherker *et al.*, 2005), New Zealand (Chalmers *et al.*, 1996) and Canada (Laforest *et al.*, 2001) suggest that falls of 1.5–2 m or above cause more frequent and serious injuries. The specification of a 'safe' height will always be contentious, but these data indicate that a maximum equipment height of 1.5 m is appropriate for standard playground settings.

Infrastructure interventions that promote safety
As well as focusing on particular measures that aim to reduce the incidence, severity or risk of specific types of injury, policy-makers need to take strategic action that will nurture and facilitate the planning, implementation and evaluation of such measures. This strategic action includes population-wide planning, the identification of strong leadership, the establishment of surveillance systems, the creation of national or local focal points, enhancing capacity through skills training and the investment of resources in research.

► PRACTICE NUGGET

Policy-makers need to take strategic action that will nurture and facilitate the planning, implementation and evaluation of injury prevention measures. This includes:
- population-wide planning;
- the identification of strong leadership;
- the establishment of surveillance systems;
- the creation of national or local focal points;
- enhancing capacity through skills training;
- investment of resources in research.

Develop comprehensive population-wide safety strategies and implementation plans
The adoption of a comprehensive, strategic, population-wide approach to injury prevention is the most fundamental infrastructural requirement. A necessary, although in itself insufficient, first step is to recognise injury as a public health problem. Even in countries where numerous national policies and strategies relevant to injury prevention and safety are already in place, few attempts are made to link them into a single, overarching strategic framework for safety at either national or local level. The separation, for policy purposes, of injuries into unintentional and intentional categories can lead to a failure to recognise causes, consequences and countermeasures that are common to both.

The absence of 'joined-up thinking' in this field is extremely common and produces duplication, gaps, inconsistencies, dilution of effort, impaired effectiveness and the inefficient use of resources. The WHO has repeatedly called on national governments to adopt an overall strategy for tackling all forms of injury, whether intentional or unintentional, in an integrated, coordinated manner. Although convincing data are sparse, there is some evidence that countries (such as Sweden) that demonstrate strong leadership in injury prevention combined with a commitment to multisectoral, comprehensive and integrated strategies have achieved greater progress in promoting safety than those opting for a piecemeal approach. The same arguments apply to regional or local agencies.

► LEARNING POINT

There is evidence that countries that demonstrate strong leadership in injury prevention combined with a commitment to multisectoral, comprehensive and integrated strategies have achieved greater progress in promoting safety than those opting for a piecemeal approach.

Identify strong leadership for developing vision, direction and integration
By its nature, responsibility for injury prevention and safety is distributed across many agencies both within and outside government. That diffusion of responsibility has two possible – and sometimes simultaneous – consequences. Either injury

prevention is perceived as 'everyone's business and no-one's responsibility', with the result that new initiatives are rare or non-existent, or it causes 'turf wars' between competing groups and organisations, each of which may feel that the lead role for safety should lie with them. Interagency rivalries and conflicting departmental cultures can thus pose serious barriers to cooperation and integration.

HEATED DEBATE No. 7:
Who should lead injury prevention policy and practice?

Injury prevention tends to suffer from a lack of leadership. Although a multi-agency approach is necessary, ensuring integration and avoiding duplication requires that a single agency or department, with a named individual, has the remit for leading the entire effort. That may seem an uncontroversial idea, yet it is fraught with difficulties. Who should take the lead? Will extra resources be allocated to this leadership function? What are the managerial relationships between the lead department or individual and the rest of the organisation? How will conflicting objectives or methods be resolved? Are the relevant leadership skills sufficiently available to fulfil the role?

Some argue that it scarcely matters who takes the lead for injury prevention in an organisation. On the other hand, sustained commitment to leadership is unlikely to survive unless a case can be made for a particular official or department. The growing 'community safety' movement, for example, is often led by police forces or criminal justice systems, and that may be appropriate. Alternatively, local authority or community planning partnerships may seize the initiative in response to public demands to create a safer environment, and that too can offer a viable model. By contrast, healthcare officials may be reluctant to become involved in a field to which they may feel, with some justification, that they have relatively little to contribute in a preventive sense.

Conclusion
No single agency, department or individual has an exclusive claim to leadership in injury prevention. The unavoidable reality, however, is that every serious injury, wherever it originates, exacts a cost on the healthcare system, whether in primary, secondary or tertiary care. This final common pathway is undeniable. Logic dictates, therefore, that leadership of and advocacy for this multi-agency activity should be forthcoming from the health (particularly public health) sector at both health local health authority and government level. At the same time, the complex multi-agency and multidisciplinary nature of injury prevention, particularly in relation to the planning and implementation of countermeasures, demands a sensitive, inclusive and partnership approach.

Improve national, regional and local injury data collection, dissemination and use
In clinical practice, it is axiomatic that diagnosis should precede treatment. In public health terms, a community diagnosis based on good-quality routine incidence, mortality and morbidity statistics, is equally important. At the same time, the mantra of 'more data' should not be repeated uncritically; even where high-quality data exist, the public health response may be weak. Rightly or wrongly, adequate injury surveillance is widely regarded as a prerequisite for the design and evaluation of countermeasures.

◀ LEARNING POINT ▶ ─────────────────────────────

The mantra of 'more data' should not be repeated uncritically. Even where high-quality data exist, the public health response may be weak.
● ●

Virtually no injury incidence (as opposed to mortality or healthcare usage) data are currently collected in most countries or districts, although the potential for recording presentations at emergency departments is enormous and has recently been greatly enhanced by the development of highly sophisticated patient information systems such as the Australian EDIS (Emergency Department Information System) suite of software programmes. Although EDIS contains a minimum data set for injury surveillance, its non-mandatory application will undermine the prospects for nationwide implementation. Alternative strategies involving, for example, periodic sampling of cases in time or place may therefore prove more productive and efficient (Morrison and Stone, 1998).

Create a focal point to plan, implement and evaluate safety measures

The capacity to identify, integrate and coordinate strategies and policies across the entire injury prevention and safety field is dependent on the existence or otherwise of a mechanism for focusing attention more effectively on the problem. Leadership and coordination have already been highlighted, but that may prove difficult to sustain in the long term.

One solution that has been adopted successfully in several countries (e.g. the USA, Sweden, Israel, New Zealand and Australia) is the creation of an injury prevention centre that brings together a critical mass of expertise and resources to facilitate the planning, implementation and evaluation of interventions. These centres operate on different models. They all, however, tend to have a national, regional or local remit for surveillance, training, information, prevention, monitoring and research. Initial start-up costs may be high, although longer term support may be secured thereafter through grants and sponsorship. The British Medical Association (2001) has endorsed calls for the creation of such a centre in the UK, although, so far, without success.

Enhance the capacity and infrastructure for injury prevention

Effective injury prevention demands the application of specialised skills that are in short supply in most countries. Within the healthcare system, already overstretched primary care staff (especially public health nurses or health visitors) are encouraged or expected to offer safety advice to families during routine consultations with minimal additional time and resources. Even more serious is the paucity of skill development. The training of healthcare professionals in injury prevention is patchy or entirely absent. Multidisciplinary educational programmes and training schemes need to be introduced to nurture a skilled workforce able to champion, coordinate and implement action throughout the country. In parallel, administrative structures should be established or adapted to ensure the effective deployment of skills and resources nationally, regionally and locally. Put bluntly, there is no point in equipping professionals with injury prevention skills, however impressive, if there are no employment or promotion prospects for them on completion of their training.

Allocate resources for undertaking research, development, monitoring and evaluation
The generation of knowledge through high-quality epidemiological and evaluational research is the foundation for all public health. In most countries, despite the heavy burden of injuries on the health of the population, the resources allocated to injury prevention activities and research at national and local level remain miserly relative to those for other conditions such as cancer, cardiovascular and even infectious diseases. Data from the UK Clinical Research Collaboration, quoted by Nicholl (2006), show just how poorly supported injury research is.

◄ LEARNING POINT ►

Despite the heavy burden of injuries on the health of the population, the resources allocated to injury prevention activities and research at national and local level remain miserly relative to those for other conditions such as cancer, cardiovascular and infectious diseases.

Decision-making about resource allocation occurs largely at the centre and is informed by political realities. Injury (apart from suicide) is seldom an explicit health improvement priority for governments, although the term 'safety' or 'safe' often regularly appears in strategic policy statements. Because these terms tend to have criminal justice rather than health connotations, their relevance to injury prevention may be overlooked. Moreover, the connections between injuries and other public health topics may pass unnoticed. All anti-obesity strategies, for example, emphasise the importance of encouraging more exercise in children, and that, in turn, may inadvertently increase injury risk. These observations require translation into national and local action in terms of research, policy development, monitoring and evaluation.

Another important element of the safety infrastructure is a well-organised trauma care system (see Chapter 8).

SUMMARY OF CHAPTER 6

Implementing unintentional injury prevention

What works in unintentional child injury prevention:

Interventions that reduce injury incidence, severity or risk – roads
- Apply area-wide urban safety measures.
- Promote average traffic speed reduction in both residential and rural areas.
- Improve enforcement of seat belt/child restraint legislation.
- Encourage universal bicycle/motorcycle helmet wearing.
- Facilitate modifications to vehicle design.
- Implement community-based education/advocacy measures to protect pedestrians.

Interventions that reduce injury incidence, severity or risk – homes
- Promote use of child-resistant closures and packaging.
- Provide, distribute, install and maintain smoke detectors/alarms/sprinklers.
- Ensure a safe temperature of domestic hot water via thermostatic mixing valves.
- Install window safety mechanisms to prevent falls from heights.
- Encourage the installation of stair gates at the tops of stairs.
- Implement parenting support/early intervention home visiting programmes.
- Seek to eliminate or modify baby walkers.
- Seek to eliminate or modify cigarette lighters and cigarettes (self-extinguishing).
- Promote the sale and wearing of non-flamable sleepwear.

Interventions that reduce injury incidence, severity or risk – elsewhere
- Promote the use of personal flotation devices for water recreation.
- Increase the presence of adequately trained lifeguards at water recreational facilities.
- Seek the implementation of isolation fencing around private swimming pools.
- Construct energy-absorbent surfaces in playgrounds.
- Install playground equipment of an appropriate height (1.5 m for young children).

Infrastructure interventions that promote safety
- Develop comprehensive population-wide safety strategies and implementation plans.
- Identify strong leadership for developing vision, direction and integration.
- Improve national, regional and local injury data collection, dissemination and use.
- Create a focal point to plan, implement and evaluate safety measures.
- Enhance the capacity and infrastructure for injury prevention.
- Allocate resources for undertaking research, development, monitoring and evaluation.

CHAPTER 7

Implementing intentional injury prevention

Learning objectives

■ To have a basic knowledge of the evidence on the efficacy of measures designed to prevent intentional injuries

■ To be aware of the growing research evidence relating to the prevention of interpersonal violence

■ To understand the nature of the public health response to violence against children

■ To be aware of recent thinking on how collective violence might be prevented

Prevention of suicide and deliberate self-harm

Several countries have developed national suicide prevention strategies, with results that are unclear or difficult to evaluate. Interventions range from social or environmental measures (e.g. reducing the availability or lethality of suicide means such as firearms) to individually targeted ones (e.g. to reverse suicidal ideation), with a strong bias in favour of the latter. Suicide prevention has tended to be regarded as falling within the remit of the mental health sector in most countries, with a reliance on psychological screening and case finding, although that view may be slowly changing. In 2001, the US Department of Health and Human Services (Department of Health and Human Services, 2001) published a comprehensive National Strategy for Suicide Prevention that adopted a community-wide approach embracing public health as well as clinical measures. This resonates well with World Health Organization (WHO) calls for a multisectoral approach within the broader context of injury prevention.

A systematic review of suicide prevention interventions (Guo and Harstall, 2004) classified the various approaches as follows:

❑ prevention (universal or selective);
❑ treatment (case identification and treatment);
❑ maintenance (long-term care and follow-up).

The authors noted that over half of the 30 interventions evaluated could be described as treatment rather than prevention or maintenance. Of the programmes aimed at children, only school-based interventions aimed at adolescents (12–19 years) based on behaviour change and coping strategies appeared to be effective. In high-risk adolescents, social support and skill development appeared to reduce risk and enhance protection. In patients who had already self-harmed, a range of psychological and pharmacological interventions appeared to offer some benefit.

■ LEARNING POINT

Suicide prevention in children has rarely been evaluated. Most studies have focused on clinical treatment rather than primary prevention.

■ PRACTICE NUGGET

Effective child and adolescent suicide prevention includes:
- school-based interventions aimed at adolescents (12–19 years of age) based on behavioural change and coping strategies;
- physician education in suicide recognition and treatment;
- restriction of access to lethal suicide means.

Another systematic review (Mann *et al.*, 2005), involving an examination of research findings by suicide experts from 15 countries, concluded that only two interventions were supported by evidence: education of physicians in the recognition and treatment of depression (with an important caveat that the use of selective serotonin reuptake inhibitors in children required further study), and restriction of access to lethal means (e.g. firearm control, detoxification of domestic gas and use of blister packs for medicines).

In summary, there is a paucity of high-quality evaluation studies of suicide-preventive measures. Most of the interventions that have been studied adopt a highly targeted, clinical perspective rather than a total-population preventive one. The only interventions that have clearly been shown to be effective in reducing suicide rates in younger age groups are school-based interventions aimed at adolescents, physician education in suicide recognition and treatment, and restriction of access to lethal suicide means. In the future, governments and professionals will need to undertake more long-term strategic thinking in addressing the global challenge of suicide and deliberate self-harm (DSH). This will involve adopting an explicitly public health approach spanning the entire life cycle, including the early years.

Prevention of deliberate self-harm

From a public health perspective, primary preventive approaches include early interventions such as parenting support and the nurturing of emotionally healthy school environments. The availability of counselling and clinical services for adolescents may help deflect some children from a trajectory that leads to DSH. And good-quality post-incident care can fulfil a tertiary preventive function. In most cases, DSH is neither a reflection of suicidal ideas nor a precursor of a serious suicide attempt. Nevertheless, services can intervene constructively to prevent further harm with counselling and other forms of therapy if these are made available through confidential telephone helplines (e.g. ChildLine and There4me in the UK) or other non-threatening, non-judgemental and non-stigmatising channels.

■ LEARNING POINT

In most cases, DSH in children and adolescents is neither a reflection of suicidal ideas nor a precursor of a serious suicide attempt.

Prevention of interpersonal violence

The public health approach to violence requires a paradigm shift away from viewing it as a consequence of 'criminal behaviour' in individuals towards overlapping 'pathological processes' in individuals, families, communities and society as a whole (the social ecological model). A systematic, population-based approach to action involves taking these steps: defining the problem, identifying causes, developing an evidence-based response, and evaluating its impact.

To prevent violence, early (0–3 years) intervention could hold the key. As a form of primary prevention, supporting parents in developing attunement with their infants may be the most cost-effective approach. Hosking and Walsh (2005) argue that the 'trigger' factors, such as poverty and alcohol misuse, are extremely difficult to influence over reasonably short timescales and that our main efforts should be directed at individual propensity. In other words, we need to stop manufacturing human 'bombs'.

■ LEARNING POINT

The public health approach to violence requires a paradigm shift away from viewing it as a form of individual 'criminal behaviour' towards 'pathological processes' in individuals, families, communities and society as a whole.

Detection and management of child maltreatment

Healthcare professionals face almost insoluble dilemmas in trying to distinguish unintentional child injuries from abuse or neglect. This is illustrated by the example of burns and scalds in pre-school children. These are among the most common injuries presenting to emergency departments (EDs), and most are unintentional. A minority are, however, the result of abuse or neglect, and diagnostic misclassification is probably a frequent occurrence, particularly in children who repeatedly present to EDs with apparently unintentional injuries.

One (albeit indirect) way of testing the misclassification hypothesis is to follow up 'unintentional' injuries and observe longer term outcomes. A study in Wales

(James-Ellison *et al.*, 2009) reported that young children who presented with burns were more likely to be subsequently referred to social services than matched controls. The authors postulated that abuse and (especially) neglect is underdiagnosed in children presenting with burn injuries, and that these injuries could be used as surrogate markers indicating a need for closer supervision and follow-up by professionals.

The UK National Institute for Health and Clinical Excellence (NICE; 2009) has issued clinical guidance to healthcare professionals on when to suspect possible child maltreatment. It was issued as a result of the perceived failings of the UK National Health Service and other agencies in detecting and intervening in high-profile cases of maltreatment such as those of Victoria Climbié and 'Baby Peter'. The guidance places much emphasis on effective and sensitive communication – with the child, the parents or carers and colleagues – and suggests a logical stepwise approach that may be summarised as:

- ❑ consider the possibility of maltreatment;
- ❑ suspect and refer when appropriate;
- ❑ exclude maltreatment only if a convincing alternative explanation is found;
- ❑ record all observations, views and actions throughout the process.

A summary version of the guideline is shown in Figure 7.1.

The problem of child maltreatment is frequently articulated exclusively in terms of the role of statutory agencies in 'child protection' – meaning the diagnosis and recording of abuse by social workers and clinicians followed by the implementation of a procedural protocol for holding a multidisciplinary case conference, placing the child on a child protection register, monitoring the family, removing (if necessary) the child, and triggering a criminal investigation. Child protection or 'safeguarding' procedures are becoming increasingly tightly defined within the various legal jurisdictions in the UK. All professionals who have responsibilities for or contact with children or their parents (or carers) are expected to know with whom to raise concerns about possible abuse, and when and how to make a referral to a local authority social services department or the police. Detailed guidance for professionals is available on the National Society for the Prevention of Cruelty to Children website (www.nspcc.org.uk/Inform/research/questions/reporting_child_abuse_wda74908.html accessed 7 February 2011).

There is no denying that child abuse is an extremely distressing phenomenon for all who encounter it, as either victims or professionals. Knowledge is, however, rapidly being disseminated, and there is enormous scope for better training and skills development among front-line professionals. Adopting a holistic approach, in which the entire family and its internal dynamics is considered, is likely to raise awareness of the possibility of abuse. Developing effective interventions is likely to prove enormously challenging – hence the importance of primary prevention.

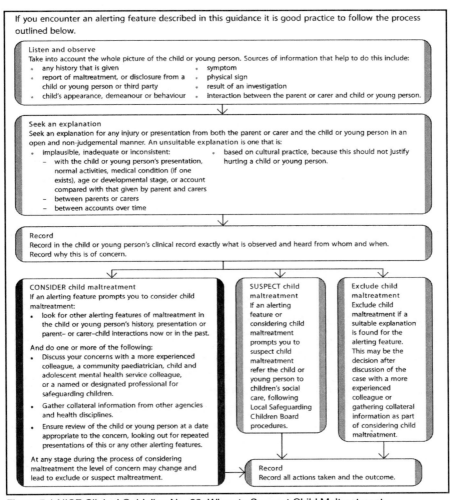

Figure 7.1 NICE Clinical Guideline No. 89: When to Suspect Child Maltreatment.
Source: www.nice.org.uk/nicemedia/live/12183/44872/44872.pdf (accessed 7 February 2011). Reproduced by kind permission of the WHO.

■ PRACTICE NUGGET

To improve the clinical detection of child maltreatment, adopt a logical stepwise approach:

■ Consider the possibility of maltreatment.

■ Suspect and refer when appropriate.

■ Exclude maltreatment only if a convincing alternative explanation is found.

■ Record all observations, views and actions throughout the process.

Nevertheless, high-quality clinical and social care of individual children and families, rooted in evidence-based practice guidelines (National Institute for Health and Clinical Excellence, 2009), will almost certainly contribute to improved outcomes for abused children.

Unfortunately, much of the professional, political and public response to child maltreatment has been emotive, irrational, short-term and ineffective. On each occasion when a particularly serious case comes to light, the spotlight is shone upon the agencies and professionals who are deemed to have failed the child rather than on the causes and prevention of the abuse itself. By contrast, the public health approach (when it is applied at all) is more circumspect, upstream and evidence-based.

■ LEARNING POINT

Child maltreatment, in the form of abuse and neglect, is underdiagnosed in children. Some experts argue that 'unintentional' injuries such as burns or scalds should be used as surrogate markers indicating a need for follow-up by professionals.

The public health response to violence against children

All governments are highly sensitive to public concerns about violence and include an array of anti-violence measures in their policy plans. These are overwhelmingly focused on the criminal justice system and on the perceived need to identify, apprehend and convict violent criminals. This reaction is akin to trying to combat defective plumbing with a floor mop rather than by repairing the leaking pipe.

Christoffel and Gallagher (2006) argue that violence is amenable to a public health approach. Notwithstanding the paucity of research data, they propose six evidence-based components as part of a comprehensive homicide and violence prevention strategy. These are: increase spending on social support (early interventions), limit alcohol consumption, restrict access to and lethality of firearms, reduce access to media violence, adopt a developmental approach emphasising positive role models, and reduce bullying behaviour, starting with younger age groups.

Using the social ecological model as a template, McVeigh et al. (2005) suggest the following action points:

- ❑ Individual level:
  - ○ Reduce unwanted pregnancies.
  - ○ Increase access to prenatal/postnatal services.
  - ○ Provide child maltreatment programmes.
  - ○ Provide social development training.
  - ○ Provide academic enrichment programmes.
- ❑ Relationship level:
  - ○ Provide home visiting services.
  - ○ Provide parenting programmes.

- ○ Provide anti-bullying programmes.
- ○ Provide mentoring services.
- ❑ *Community level*:
  - ○ Train professionals in the screening, detection and referral of victims of violence.
  - ○ Change the school culture of institutions (schools, care homes, etc.).
  - ○ Provide coordinated community interventions.
  - ○ Disrupt illegal weapon markets.
  - ○ Implement alcohol/drug reduction strategies.
- ❑ *Societal level*:
  - ○ De-concentrate poverty and reduce inequality.
  - ○ Strengthen the police and judicial system.
  - ○ Reduce media violence.

◖PRACTICE NUGGET◗

US-based writers Christoffel and Gallagher (2006) propose the following components for a homicide and violence prevention strategy:
- ■ Increase spending on social support (early interventions).
- ■ Limit alcohol consumption.
- ■ Restrict access to and lethality of firearms.
- ■ Reduce access to media violence.
- ■ Adopt a developmental approach emphasising positive role models.
- ■ Reduce bullying behaviour, starting with younger age groups.

Screening for child abuse

The healthcare sector has a particular responsibility to identify and protect children from abuse. Attempts have been made to establish screening programmes, usually based at EDs, to detect abuse and limit its damage. Assuming that most children suffering abuse will present at EDs, this seems a rational approach provided that the principles of screening, and its evaluation, are borne in mind (see Chapter 4). Although around 2–10% of all presentations at EDs are estimated to be due to abuse, detection rates are notoriously low. This has led to the introduction of clinical protocols in an effort to improve detection through screening without generating too many false-positive results. A systematic review of reports of interventions designed to increase the detection rate of abuse (Louwers *et al.*, 2010) identified only four appropriate papers. The rate of detection, as indicated by the weighted mean of three studies, increased by 180%, but the detection rate of confirmed cases (reported in only two studies) did not increase. The authors concluded that the available evidence is insufficient to support screening and called for further studies to be performed.

LEARNING POINT

Attempts have been made to establish screening programmes, usually based at EDs, to detect child abuse and limit its damage. The available evidence appears insufficient to support screening.

• •

In reviewing the research evidence on violence prevention, the WHO, in conjunction with Liverpool John Moores University (World Health Organization/John Moores University, 2009), identified seven key strategies that overlap with those proposed by Christoffel and Gallagher (2006):

❏ developing safe, stable and nurturing relationships between children and their parents and caregivers;

❏ developing life skills in children and adolescents;

❏ reducing the availability and harmful use of alcohol;

❏ reducing access to guns, knives and pesticides;

❏ promoting gender equality to prevent violence against women;

❏ changing cultural and social norms that support violence;

❏ victim identification, care and support programmes.

Only the first of these appears to prevent child maltreatment, although there is good evidence that the second may prevent youth violence. Early interventions such as the home-visitation-based Nurse–Family Partnership (Olds and Henderson, 1986) and the centre-based Positive Parenting Programme (Sanders, 2008) have been claimed to reduce the incidence of child maltreatment (Prinz *et al.*, 2009) and may improve child behaviour as well as reduce the incidence of other long-term negative outcomes, including violence. Social development programmes (which are designed to boost emotional behavioural and social competencies) may prevent youth violence. Pre-school enrichment programmes (which provide children with academic and social skills at an early age) appear promising. These interventions have, however, been mainly evaluated to date in high-income countries.

HEATED DEBATE No 8: Should we ban corporal punishment?

Although the UN Convention on the Rights of the Child forbids corporal punishment, it remains widely used throughout the world. Few aspects of child-rearing provoke such controversy. Many otherwise mild-mannered parents regard the physical punishment of children, sometimes involving the use of an implement such as a slipper, leather belt or stick, as perfectly reasonable and acceptable, and deeply resent any attempt by governments to legislate or even to issue guidelines as an intrusion on their human rights. Others defend the practice of hitting children ('lovingly') with the bare hand as justifiable as a means of behavioural discipline and even of promoting safety despite both the moral counterarguments and the lack of evidence of its effectiveness.

Opponents of corporal punishment emphasise the double standard whereby adults have legal protection against assault while children do not. Furthermore, they point to the research evidence that some adults seem liable to cross the line from chastisement to abuse, and to the role of legal sanctions in acting as a deterrent. Several studies have demonstrated an association between the use of physical punishment and unequivocal child abuse (Zolotor *et al.*, 2008). Perpetrators of abuse regularly claim that their abusive behaviour started as 'normal' punishment that subsequently escalated.

The historical experience of Sweden is instructive in this regard. In the 19th and early 20th centuries, corporal punishment was common in that county, with many children experiencing severe beatings. In response to growing public debate, the practice was outlawed in the gymnasium (secondary school) system in 1928, and by the 1960s its legal defence was removed in all other settings as well. Public opinion and legal practice tended to lag behind the legislation, however, and some ambiguity remained over whether the law banned or merely disapproved of corporal punishment. In 1978, the Parents' Code was amended to clarify the position, and the practice was banned – although without legal sanction in the form of penalties. This avoided criminalising parents, altered public attitudes and offered opportunities for early intervention with troubled families.

Since then, large-scale public education campaigns about the new law have been mounted and discussed in schools and parent education classes. There has been a strong emphasis on non-violent alternatives that parents can use to maintain discipline. Surveys have shown that Swedish parents overwhelmingly support the law, and rates of severe child abuse have declined steeply. Several other countries, in Scandinavia and elsewhere, have followed suit. The UK has passed legislation outlawing the use of implements but has stopped short of a full-scale ban.

Conclusion
Most forms of corporal punishment are probably relatively harmless and cause only transient pain or discomfort. Nevertheless, a minority of adults cross the line from reasonable punishment to outright abuse. As we have no methods of identifying and deterring such adults, the safest course would seem to be to outlaw the practice altogether while offering evidence-based alternative methods of maintaining discipline. Countries that have gone down this road have reported much reduced levels of severe child maltreatment as a consequence of banning 'mild' maltreatment, with no obvious adverse emotional, educational or social consequences. In any case, most of the argument is now irrelevant following the international consensus that developed around the writing and implementation of the UN Convention on the Rights of the Child. As well as being ineffective and potentially harmful, corporal punishment is now widely regarded as immoral and illegal.

How can collective violence be prevented?
A multi-pronged approach to reduce the incidence of collective violence needs to take account of the modifiability of risk factors, the international organisational and legal context, the state of public opinion, the role of the health sector, and the importance of careful documentation and research. Because of the paucity of research, the evidence base for these measures is extremely limited. Moreover, experience has shown that cynical political calculations by individual countries, groups of countries or leaders tend to trump proposals for countermeasures that are motivated by humanitarian concerns.

Krug *et al.* (2002), writing for the WHO, documented the wide range of adverse consequences of collective violence, including war, terrorism and torture, on population health. They suggested several strategies for preventing collective violence, including reducing its potential by modifying risk factors, promoting the compliance of countries with international agreements, responding quickly and effectively to outbreaks of collective violence through political and humanitarian action, deploying peace keeping measures by the United Nations (UN) in conflict zones, harnessing the influence of the healthcare sector to document and respond to violence, and carefully recording and disseminating information, including that generated by research, on violent conflicts around the world. Two of these strategies are described in more detail below.

◀ PRACTICE NUGGET

To prevent violent conflict, several simultaneous strategies are necessary:
- modifying risk factors for collective violence;
- promoting the compliance of countries with international agreements;
- responding quickly and effectively to outbreaks of collective violence through political and humanitarian action;
- deploying peace-keeping measures by the UN in conflict zones;
- harnessing the influence of the healthcare sector to document and respond to violence;
- carefully recording and disseminating information, including that generated by research.

Risk factor modification

Among the key national policies required to minimise the risk of collective violence within or between countries and communities are to:
- ❑ reduce poverty, in both absolute and relative terms, and ensure that development assistance is targeted so as to make the greatest possible impact on poverty;
- ❑ make decision-making more accountable;
- ❑ reduce social and other forms of inequality;
- ❑ reduce access to biological, chemical, nuclear and other weapons.

Promotion of compliance with international agreements

A key strategy for preventing violent conflict is to seek to promote and apply internationally agreed treaties, including those relating to human rights. National governments can play their part by upholding the spirit of the Charter of the United Nations, which calls for the prevention of aggression and the promotion of international peace and security. Furthermore, they have an obligation to adhere to international legal instruments including the 1949 Geneva Conventions and their 1977 Additional Protocols.

A permanent mechanism now exists, in the form of the International Criminal Court, to deal with genocide, war crimes and crimes against humanity. It will also presumably act as deterrent against violence directed at civilian populations. Unfortunately, the application of these various agreements is subject to international political processes that may sometimes be unhelpful. Member states on international bodies such as the United Nations Security Council and related committees may fail to act appropriately or may adopt biased postures. This behaviour merely undermines the intentions of international treaties by perverting the processes for cynical political reasons.

◖LEARNING POINT◗

A key strategy for preventing violent conflict is to seek to promote and apply internationally agreed treaties, including those relating to human rights. A permanent mechanism now exists, in the form of the International Criminal Court, to deal with genocide, war crimes and crimes against humanity.

HEATED DEBATE No 9: To intervene militarily or not?

Most pacifists unconditionally oppose any form of military action, whether in self-defence or for any other reason, however 'just'. That is an entrenched, and often religiously inspired, moral position that should be respected but cannot easily be addressed through argument and debate.

The non-pacifist majority is bound to confront harder choices. Is military intervention justified, not just in self-defence of the communities within which we live, but also to protect others living in foreign parts from harm? Arbor (2008) highlights a dilemma that faces contemporary foreign policy-makers in the wake of recent controversial military interventions in Iraq and Afghanistan. On the one hand, going to war is unappetising, hazardous for the combatants and for civilians, unpredictable in terms of the outcome and often politically unpopular. On the other, a refusal to intervene with force may result in large numbers of avoidable deaths and injuries inflicted on innocent populations by the unrestrained violence of brutal regimes. Is there an internationally recognised means of resolving this thorny issue?

The short answer is no. War, even when it is perceived to be just or necessary, will always provoke heated responses on either side of the argument. At the extreme poles will be found pacifists and militarists. Neither is likely to be able to contribute constructively to rational debate. Closer to the centre will lie a range of views, many of which appear irreconcilable. Advocates will claim that war is the lesser of two evils, while opponents will deny the validity of legitimate *casus belli*. Both will assume the mantle of moral and legal superiority.

The mantra of many anti-war campaigners that the allied invasion of Iraq in 2003 was 'immoral and illegal' is hard to challenge objectively. The morality or otherwise of a military conflict is always a matter of subjective judgement, while a ruling on legality can only be assessed by recourse to an accepted legal authority. Selective and often tendentious citing of the UN Charter tends to generate more heat than light. It is salutary to recall that interventions to try to end large-scale atrocities such as those perpetrated by the Khmer

Rouge regime in Cambodia were frequently condemned as illegal violations of national sovereignty as they were not explicitly mandated by the UN Security Council.

The collective global failure to prevent genocide in the former Yugoslavia, Rwanda and Darfur, led to a reassessment of and a change in international law. In 2005, the Summit of the world's leaders endorsed the new principle of the 'responsibility to protect' populations – such as those being subjected to genocidal attack by their own government in pre-2003 Iraq and elsewhere – from gross human rights violations. This overturned the previous norm of non-interference. Critics were quick to cite this development as a form of 'moral imperialism', while Arbor argues that the new doctrine holds enormous promise for the protective reach of the UN and other agencies.

Conclusion
War is clearly always undesirable yet arguably sometimes necessary. The success or failure of military intervention will depend – as in all areas of international law – on the both the sound political judgement of individual leaders and the collective will of the international community as expressed through the UN Security Council. Unfortunately, with rare exceptions, historical experience is hardly encouraging.

Combating political violence and terrorism

There is a further obstacle to the deployment of international treaties or other forms of concerted political action as a means of preventing conflict. A fluctuating number of violent incidents around the world is attributable to the activities of non-state actors whose aims, psychology, methods and organisation are obscure or constantly changing. These groups are often described as terrorists, although there is no agreed definition of terrorism. One definition is that terrorism involves the use of methods designed to inflict death, injury and overwhelming fear on civilians rather than military personnel, and in an area wider than that of the military target itself. Another is that terrorism is simply any 'politically motivated violence or the threat of violence, especially against civilians, with the intent to instil fear' (Sidel and Levy, 2009).

◀ LEARNING POINT

Terrorism may be defined as any 'politically motivated violence or the threat of violence, especially against civilians, with the intent to instil fear'.

Politically motivated violence is far from new but came under the media spotlight in the 1970s in conflict zones as far apart as South America, Africa, the Middle East and Northern Ireland. Terrorism may be a tactic in wars occurring between states, within a state (civil war) or in insurgencies. The financing, training and arming of terrorist or paramilitary groups may be difficult to ascertain as they may be used as proxies for larger geopolitical disputes (e.g. during the Cold War). The members of such groups tend to portray themselves as 'freedom fighters' struggling against injustice and oppression, and, in some cases, have succeeded in rallying to their support politicians, intellectuals, academics and professionals who are seduced by the sanitised language of 'guerrilla warfare', 'armed struggle', 'resistance' and 'anti-imperialism'. Blame for civilian casualties is invariably allotted to the alleged crimes of their adversaries rather than to their own actions. The most notorious act of mass terrorism of modern times was the attack on the World Trade Center in New York and the Pentagon in Washington, DC, on 11 September 2001 perpetrated by Al Qaeda, killing around 3,000 people, most of whom were civilians.

Although terrorists are often described in pursuing the tactics of 'asymmetric warfare' (a term implying that the resources available to them are few in comparison with those at the disposal of their targets), they may nevertheless achieve a high level of sophistication in their exploitation of globalised information and communication technology, arms markets and theatres of operation. Unlike conventional armies, they are seldom identifiable by the wearing of uniforms or by the use of detectable lines of command and control. They use weaponry of all kinds, including weapons of mass destruction, are capable of extreme and sustained violence against real or imagined enemies, are frequently motivated by political or religious fanaticism, may be undeterred by the threat of military or economic responses from states or international organisations, and ignore legal codes of conduct such as the Geneva Convention.

Preventing mass terrorism is extremely problematic for several reasons. First, too little knowledge is available about the structure, operation, motivation or whereabouts of these groups. Second, they may receive powerful political, diplomatic, economic and military support from states, organisations or individuals in ways that are undetectable. Third, they may obtain tacit support from third parties who hold uninformed or partisan views on the 'root causes' of this type of violence, its expression and nature, and of the most appropriate means of confronting it. Apart from adopting the basic conceptual principles that apply to all types of violence prevention, the range of evidence-based measures for intervening to prevent terrorism at its source (primary prevention), as opposed to interrupting the activities and effectiveness of terrorist groups (secondary prevention), remains limited.

Governments, international bodies and counterterrorism agencies have tried to adopt a multi-pronged approach to the prevention of terrorism including military, judicial, political and social components. The European Council, for example, following the atrocities committed in Madrid in 2004, called for a European-wide anti-terrorism strategy comprising a tightening of international legal enforcement, better cross-border policing and cooperation, and more effective intelligence. The European Union (EU) Plan to Combat Terrorism had the following high-level objectives (www.consilium.europa.eu/uedocs/cmsUpload/79635.pdf accessed 7 February 2011):

- ❏ Deepen the international consensus and enhance international efforts to combat terrorism.
- ❏ Reduce the access of terrorists to financial and other economic resources.
- ❏ Maximise capacity within EU bodies and Member States to detect, investigate and prosecute terrorists and prevent terrorist attacks.
- ❏ Protect the security of international transport and ensure effective systems of border control.
- ❏ Enhance the capability of Member States to deal with the consequences of a terrorist attack.
- ❏ Address the factors that contribute to support for, and recruitment into, terrorism.
- ❏ Target actions under EU external relations towards priority Third Countries where counter-terrorist capacity or commitment to combating terrorism needs to be enhanced.

Counterterrorism strategies of this kind are challenging to implement. Measures designed to increase intelligence and improve security may be perceived to be controversial and even to conflict with human rights. Some non-governmental organisations (NGOs), including Amnesty International, call for a purely law enforcement response to terrorism despite the practical and legal obstacles. This has led some countries to pass emergency antiterrorist legislation (e.g. the UK Prevention of Terrorism Act) to enhance the capacity of the security services to monitor, arrest and detain suspects. Others emphasise the need for stringent and sometimes pre-emptive policing military measures. These are not mutually exclusive approaches, and the balance is a fine one. In addition, evaluating success is equally problematic. The trend of fatalities and injuries from terrorist acts around the world appears to be downwards, and that may reflect a degree of success in this area. Nevertheless, the motivation and funding of extremist groups, whether on the political right or left, whether religious or nationalist, or whether a combination of some of these, remains undiminished and should not be underestimated.

◁LEARNING POINT▷───────────────────────

Counterterrorism strategies are challenging to devise and implement. Measures designed to increase intelligence and improve security may be perceived to be controversial and even to conflict with human rights.

• •

Influencing public opinion about collective violence

The globalisation of information through the 24-hour news media, the Internet and numerous social networking sites such as Facebook and Twitter has resulted in a rapid increase of awareness throughout the world about egregious military behaviour, human rights abuses and breaches of international law. This is hugely beneficial in one sense in that public opinion, either generally or operating through lobby groups, can be mobilised more easily to exert pressure on politicians to take action. On the other hand, it is a double-edged sword as sophisticated media and NGOs increasingly have the ability to disseminate both accurate and biased information with much greater effectiveness and rapidity than in the past.

Role of the health sector in preventing collective violence

The notion that the health sector has a role to play in the prevention of mass violence seems counterintuitive. Yet there are real opportunities for intervention of which healthcare professionals may be unaware. The WHO suggests some of these:

- ❑ Investing in health and social services can help to maintain social cohesion and stability.
- ❑ Identifying and remedying social inequalities in health and healthcare access can reduce tensions between social sectors of the population.
- ❑ By publicising the impact of conflicts on the health, social and economic status of the population, health workers can raise awareness among the media and decision-makers of the need for preventive action.
- ❑ The health sector can act as an early warning system for the detection of signs of impending conflict and alert partner agencies and governments.
- ❑ The efficient, effective and equitable provision and adaptation of health services to populations suffering from the effects of conflict can mitigate the physical and psychological trauma.

Not all of these actions are likely to prove effective, and the evidence base is somewhat patchy and anecdotal. Moreover, the preventive level that each represents varies: the first three of these measures are forms of primary prevention, the fourth is secondary prevention, while the last is tertiary prevention.

Surveillance, documentation and research

As in all areas of public health, surveillance and documentation is an essential prerequisite for effective action. Because the data on collective violence are so often deficient or suspect, a pragmatic approach is warranted, while always being mindful of the potentially negative consequences of misleading information. International agencies, such as the various specialised bodies of the UN, have an important role to play, as do NGOs. All have responsibilities to ensure that data are collected, analysed and disseminated as accurately and as impartially as possible.

In 2002, in response to growing public and public concern about homicide and suicide, the US Centers for Disease Control established the National Violent Death Reporting System (NVDRS). Its goal is 'to provide communities with a clearer understanding of violent deaths so they can be prevented' (www.cdc.gov/violenceprevention/nvdrs/index.html accessed 7 February 2011). The NVDRS seeks to accomplish this goal by informing decision-makers about the magnitude, trends and characteristics of violent deaths so that appropriate preventive efforts can be put in place, and by evaluating state-based preventive programmes and strategies. Its methods comprise the collection of data on violent deaths from multiple sources, including death certificates, police reports, medical examiner reports and crime laboratories.

In the UK, a surgeon, Jonathan Shepherd, formed the Violence and Society Research Group, comprising clinicians, police officers and others committed to sharing and analysing information on assaults from EDs across England and Wales (Sivarajasingam *et al.*, 2003). This work has led to interventions in assault 'hot spots' that appear to have reduced the incidence of violence. In 2000, the Group established the National Violence Surveillance Network, which monitors the incidence of assaults using data from 60 EDs throughout England and Wales.

There is a potentially huge research agenda in the field of collective violence, spanning its causes, impacts, prevention and amelioration. The public health research community has barely scratched the surface of this virtually ubiquitous and highly disturbing phenomenon.

SUMMARY OF CHAPTER 7

Implementing intentional injury prevention

Suicide

There is a paucity of high-quality evaluation studies of suicide preventive measures. Most of the interventions that have been studied adopt a highly targeted, clinical perspective rather than total-population preventive one. The only interventions that have clearly been shown to be effective in reducing suicide rates in younger age groups are:

■ school-based interventions aimed at adolescents;

■ physician education in suicide recognition and treatment;

■ restriction of access to lethal suicide means.

Deliberate self-harm

■ Primary preventive approaches to deliberate self-harm include early interventions such as parenting support and the nurturing of emotionally healthy school environments.

■ The availability of counselling and clinical services for adolescents may help deflect some children from a trajectory that leads to deliberate self-harm.

■ Good-quality post-incident care can fulfil a tertiary preventive function.

Interpersonal violence

The public health approach to violence requires a paradigm shift from viewing it as a consequence of 'criminal behaviour' in individuals towards overlapping 'pathological processes' in individuals, families, communities and society as a whole (the social ecological model). Countermeasures may then be aimed at all of these levels.

Individual level

- Reduce unwanted pregnancies.
- Increase access to prenatal/postnatal services.
- Provide child maltreatment programmes.
- Provide social development training.
- Provide academic enrichment programmes.

Relationship level

- Provide home visiting services.
- Provide parenting programmes.
- Provide anti-bullying programmes.
- Provide mentoring services.

Community level

- Train professionals in the screening, detection and referral of victims.
- Change the school culture of institutions (schools, care homes, etc.)
- Provide coordinated community interventions.
- Disrupt illegal weapon markets.
- Implement alcohol/drug reduction strategies.

Societal level

- De-concentrate poverty and reduce inequality.
- Strengthen the police and judicial system.
- Reduce media violence.

Early (0–3 years of age) intervention could hold the key to the primary prevention of violence. As a form of primary prevention, supporting parents in developing attunement with their infants may be the most cost-effective approach.

Collective violence

A multi-pronged approach is necessary to reduce the incidence of collective violence. In particular, such an approach needs to take account of:

- the modifiability of risk factors;
- the international organisational and legal context;
- the state of public opinion;
- the role of the health sector;
- the importance of careful documentation and research.

Because of the paucity of research, the evidence base for these measures is extremely limited. Nevertheless, the absence of evidence should not induce paralysis.

CHAPTER 8

Combined public health and clinical approaches to injury prevention

Learning objectives

- To understand the difference between 'horizontal' and 'vertical' interventions
- To be aware of some of the potential interventions that might achieve multiple outcomes
- To have a basic knowledge of the evidence for effective early intervention in preventing injury
- To understand the preventive role of specialist trauma care

Interventions aimed at multiple outcomes

A distinction is sometimes drawn between preventive interventions that are vertical and those that are horizontal. Vertical injury prevention interventions are fairly narrowly focused on specific injury types or locations such as roads, schools or homes. The 'low-hanging fruit' of relatively easy technical and regulatory interventions falls under this heading (Johnston, 2010). Examples include drink-driving laws and smoke detectors. Horizontal interventions address the underlying determinants of a range of injuries simultaneously. Examples of the latter include safer transport infrastructures (to protect vulnerable pedestrians as well as vehicle occupants), gun control measures (that reduce the incidence of homicide, suicide and unintentional gunshot wounds) and restricting access to potentially harmful medication (thereby reducing the incidence of suicide and unintentional poisoning). Horizontal interventions may be more ambitious still, addressing upstream determinants of injuries and other disorders by reducing exposure and enhancing resilience. A particularly striking horizontal intervention is parenting support.

Parenting and early years – the single common pathway for all types of injury

The 'early origins of disease' is a phrase that is familiar to all public health professionals. The links between intrauterine influences, in the form of either hazardous exposures (such as thalidomide) or deficiencies (such as inadequate folate), and a range of diseases in childhood and later are well established. Postnatal factors, such as breastfeeding and sleeping position, may also play a causal role in childhood mortality and morbidity. Less well known is the emerging evidence that many injuries may be traced, aetiologically, to early childhood, and that these early influences can have an impact on the risk of injury well into adult life.

Felitti *et al.* (1998) argue that their Adverse Childhood Experiences (ACE) study of 17,000 socio-economically homogeneous (middle-class) adults clearly demonstrates that early childhood trauma has profound and lifelong effects on later mental and physical health. Based on retrospective data accounts collected from study subjects, high ACE scores are strongly and positively correlated with a range of outcomes in adult life. Some of these are associated with increased injury risk – including addictions (alcohol, tobacco and drugs), obesity (a form of addiction) and depression – while others are part of the injury spectrum (violence, deliberate self-harm and suicide). The time line seems to fit with cause rather than effect (of a confounding variable), i.e. the onset of the disease outcome postdates the ACE. A retrospective study is, nevertheless, subject to bias, confounding and misclassification.

The implications of these studies are far-reaching and relate to aetiology, treatment and prevention. If the aetiological pathway is confirmed, it reinforces the case for focusing attention on the early years for a whole range of child and adult disorders, including injury of all types. And treatment strategies should be devised – and evaluated – that include an attempt to address the ongoing damage caused to the adult by the childhood trauma. Most importantly, primary prevention should seek to minimise ACEs in the population through whatever tools are available (parenting support, early years interventions, etc.). The impact of these interventions will need to be assessed over many decades. A recent systematic review (Kendrick *et al.*, 2007) indicates that parenting education and training programmes appear to reduce the risk of injuries in disadvantaged groups (see below), although that does not preclude the possibility that all children might benefit from the interventions. Whether these programmes operate through the prevention or amelioration of ACEs or as a result of more direct impacts, such as by reducing exposure to environmental hazards and by encouraging the use of safety equipment, is unclear.

ACEs are not the whole story, of course, as they will interact positively or negatively with later experiences. In the case of injury, as mentioned earlier, exacerbating or trigger factors (e.g. poverty, alcohol and environment) should also be acknowledged – the 'fuses' as well as the 'bombs', as the WAVE report (Hosking and Walsh, 2005) describes them. Both are important for primary prevention. Some of the fuses may have a similar aetiology to the bombs (e.g. alcohol and aggression).

The corollary of recognising the damaging role of ACEs is the nurturing of positive childhood experiences (parental affection, a stable family structure and non-violent methods of discipline) that could play a health-promoting (salutogenic) role in the development of resilience and the avoidance of risk-taking behaviour.

Evidence for effective early intervention

Early childhood intervention programmes, of the kind pioneered by Olds *et al.* (2004), have repeatedly been found to produce significant improvements across all domains of child development, health, education, behaviour and life success. Successful interventions adopt a two-generational approach focusing simultaneously on parents and children, and provide a combination of home visits and enriched early (pre-school) education. Most of the programmes have targeted those at highest risk, defined on the basis of social or demographic indicators.

Among the most strikingly successful programmes (Geddes *et al.*, 2010) may be counted the Nurse–Family Partnership, the High/Scope Perry Preschool Project, the Carolina Abecedarian Project, the Parents as Teachers Programme and the Incredible Years Parenting Programme. All of these have been developed in the US. The Australian Triple P and the British Sure Start initiatives have also yielded positive findings on evaluation. Moreover, economic evaluations have indicated that these interventions, while relatively expensive to implement (between $6,000 and $30,000 being spent per child or family), are highly cost-effective: every dollar invested results in returns of between around $4 and $7. These savings accrue for reductions in the use of special education facilities, fewer episodes of juvenile delinquency, fewer benefit claims and increased tax contributions.

◀ PRACTICE NUGGET ▶

Successful **parenting or early years' interventions:**
- adopt a two-generational approach;
- focus simultaneously on parents and children;
- provide a combination of home visits and enriched early (pre-school) education;
- produce a range of health benefits including lower injury rates.

To recapitulate: the ACE and other studies point to a potentially crucial role for early childhood influences on the later risk of injury. Early intervention studies point to a range of health, educational and social benefits. From a practical perspective, the key question is this: can anything be done to interrupt or modify the trajectory of child development in a way that demonstrably reduces the incidence or severity of injuries? Although the evidence remains fairly sparse, the answer appears to be yes.

In a systematic review undertaken for the Cochrane Library, Kendrick *et al.* (2007) examined 15 studies of parenting interventions, 11 of which were randomised controlled trials. The interventions were multifaceted programmes mostly comprising the home visiting of families by specially trained professionals (health visitors or public health nurses). Most of the programmes were targeted at families deemed to be at high risk of adverse health outcomes. In a meta-analysis of nine randomised controlled trials, children from the intervention families had a significantly lower (by 18%) risk of injury (risk ratio 0.82, 95% confidence interval 0.71 to 0.95) than controls. Several studies reported fewer home hazards, a home environment more conducive to child safety or a greater number of safety practices in intervention families. Parenting interventions aimed at high-risk families therefore seem to be effective in reducing the incidence of unintentional injuries in children and may promote safer home environments generally.

◾LEARNING POINT

Parenting interventions aimed at high-risk families seem to be effective in promoting home safety and reducing the incidence of unintentional injuries in children.

This is an important finding that should help guide policy-makers and practitioners. Nevertheless, several important reservations apply. First, such interventions are generally highly complex, and the mechanisms whereby they affected injury risk are unclear. Second, most are aimed at high-risk families, and doubts regularly surface (see Chapter 3) about our ability to identify, a priori, such families through routine home visiting and assessment even by trained professionals (Wright *et al.*, 2009). Third, as a consequence of the 'prevention paradox', many (probably most) injuries in the population occur in so-called low- or medium-risk families that will therefore be unaffected by targeted interventions. Finally, all of the studies included in the review were performed in high-income countries, whereas most injuries occur in low- or middle-income populations.

Role of clinicians in preventing injury

Prevention in daily clinical practice

Stone and Pearson (2009) argue that there are numerous unexploited opportunities for clinicians, including doctors, nurses and other healthcare staff involved in patient care, to become involved in injury prevention (Box 8.1). Although routine clinical work may appear to offer limited opportunities for unintentional prevention, there is growing awareness of two principles: that prevention and health promotion are core professional responsibilities of all doctors in the UK; and that all good clinical management – especially in paediatrics and trauma care – is per se a form of prevention.

Evidence on the usefulness of clinical advice to parents and children for injury prevention is conflicting. The American Academy of Pediatrics promotes a programme that appears to be highly effective and efficient – for each dollar invested, there may be a $13 return. UK researchers are more sceptical, arguing that environmental and legislative measures are likely to prove more effective. These two positions are not, however, necessarily mutually exclusive.

Box 8.1 **Five principles of injury prevention in clinical paediatric practice**

✓ Although most parents want to keep their children safe at all times, a minority do not – and the distinction between unintentional and intentional injury (abuse or neglect) is sometimes blurred.

✓ Discussing child safety with parents need not be restricted to education in the narrow sense but can include offering practical advice about legislation (e.g. on child car seat restraints) and environmental modification (e.g. the installation of a thermostatic mixing valve).

✓ Adopting an evidence-based approach as far as possible and avoiding appealing to parental 'common sense' can be misleading – many parents (wrongly) believe that cooker guards are useful and that baby walkers are safe.

✓ Promoting safety does not require 'wrapping children in cotton wool' as that would delay normal development and restrict activity, thereby increasing the risk of obesity. The aim should be to take reasonable precautions to ensure that the risk of injury to children is minimised.

✓ The nature of the risk of injury varies widely according to age and stage of development. As a rule of thumb, pre-school children are in greatest danger in the home, while school-age children face greatest risk on the roads or at play.

◀LEARNING POINT▶

Numerous unexploited opportunities exist for clinicians, including doctors, nurses and other healthcare staff involved in patient care, to become involved in injury prevention.

Clinical service development and exploitation

With a degree of imagination and initiative, paediatricians can develop and exploit existing clinical services in a way that enables them to contribute more effectively to injury prevention. Examples include:

- ❑ developing injury surveillance in accident and emergency departments, outpatient clinics and inpatient units;
- ❑ identification of children at elevated risk of injury (e.g. repeat attenders or those with substance misuse);
- ❑ encouraging the implementation or expansion of parenting interventions;
- ❑ offering explicit evidence-based advice and support to parents and carers.

The preventive role of trauma care

Trauma care – whether in the form of the initial response of the emergency services, first aid or subsequent treatment – is a form of tertiary prevention of injury. Effective intervention can take place at the scene of the incident, in hospital and following discharge, in the community. High-quality intervention by clinicians, emergency teams or even members of the general public can make a difference to an injured person's physical and psychological prognosis. Well-organised trauma response systems, including trauma centres staffed by highly trained professionals, could have a significant impact on injury mortality worldwide. Unfortunately, these are expensive to create and run. As a consequence, low- and middle-income countries struggle to provide and sustain the necessary resources to deliver such systems.

One of the simplest yet most effective immediate responses to injury is the early and skilled use of first aid. The term, which has its origins in the care of battlefield injuries in the Middle Ages, simply means the initial care provided to victims, often by members of the public rather than professionals. As defined by the UK's NHS Direct scheme, the three key aims of first aid are to preserve life, prevent further harm and promote recovery. A key first skill, which is included in the training of all emergency care practitioners, is the ABC (airways, breathing, and circulation) of resuscitation. Once the ABC has been dealt with, management may then progress to treat other non-life-threatening problems such as haemorrhage, burns and scalds, poisonings and pain.

◄ PRACTICE NUGGET

The three key **aims of first aid** are to:
- preserve life through the application of immediate ABC (airways, breathing, circulation) based resuscitation;
- prevent further harm to the injured patient;
- promote recovery following stabilisation.

First aid courses are provided by many organisations, including ambulance associations, voluntary organisations and the media. Here, for example, are two extracts from the BBC's First Aid web pages (www.bbc.co.uk/health/treatments/first_aid/index.shtml accessed 7 February 2010, and reproduced by kind permission of the BBC and British Red Cross):

FIRST AID: WHAT NOT TO DO

There are many misconceptions surrounding first aid. Below are the 'most popular' ones with details of what you should do.

Top ten first aid misconceptions

1. **You should put butter or cream on a burn.** The only thing you should put on a burn is cold water – keep the butter for cooking. Put the affected area under cold running water for at least 10 minutes.
2. **If you can't move a limb, it must be broken (or if you can move a limb, it can't be broken).** The only accurate way to diagnose a broken limb is to x-ray it.

3. **The best way to treat bleeding is to put the wound under a tap.** If you put a bleeding wound under a tap you wash away the body's clotting agents and make it bleed more, instead push on the wound.

4. **Nosebleeds are best treated by putting the head back.** If you put the head back during a nosebleed, all the blood goes down the back of the airway. Instead advise them to tilt their head forwards to allow the blood to drain out of the nostrils. Ask the person to pinch the end of their nose and breathe through their mouth.

5. **If someone has swallowed a poison you should make them sick.** If you make someone sick by putting your fingers in their mouth, the vomit may block their airway. Also if the poison burnt on the way down, it will burn on the way up. Get medical advice and if possible find out what poison was taken, at what time and how much.

6. **If you perform CPR on someone who has a pulse you can damage their heart.** The evidence is that it isn't dangerous to do chest compressions on a casualty with a pulse.

7. **You need lots of training to do first aid.** You don't – what you mostly need is common sense. You can learn enough first aid in a few minutes to save someone's life.

8. **You need lots of expensive equipment to do first aid.** You don't need any equipment to do first aid, there are lots of ways to improvise anything you need.

WHAT TO DO AT THE SCENE OF A ROAD ACCIDENT

The first person on the scene of a collision will almost certainly be another road user. So as a driver your knowledge of first aid could make a real difference to someone in the event of a road accident.

Stop. Apply handbrake. Turn off engine.

Assess conditions

○ Remain calm. Assess the scene and seriousness of the collision. Determine what happened, how many people and vehicles are involved and the exact location

Make safe

○ Make sure you stay safe: keep off the road. If you need to stop or warn approaching cars, signal to them from the pavement. Wear fluorescent reflective clothing use warning triangles, flashing lights and hazard warning lights. Don't smoke

○ If you are in a car and you come across an accident, first park safely and turn off the engine before you get out to help. Use a hazard triangle if necessary.

○ Consider the safety of others. Immobilise the vehicle/s, look out for hazards – leaking fuel, chemicals, broken glass or shed loads – guide uninjured passengers to a place of safety

Assess casualties

○ How many casualties are there? What is the severity of the injuries? Is anyone trapped? Is there a danger of fire?

Call for help

○ Dial 999 (or 112) for the emergency services. If there is no phone nearby, recruit help and send two people in opposite directions

○ Do not use mobile phones if there is a danger from petrol-spillage or fumes

Apply emergency first aid

○ Remain calm. Reassure the victims

○ Do not allow smoking or offer food or drink to casualties as this could hamper urgent medical treatment

Calling 999 (112)

Do this as soon as you can or get someone else to do it while you deal with an injured person. You will need to tell the emergency services:

○ where you are

○ what has happened (describe the accident)

○ how many people are injured

○ whether they are breathing or bleeding.

The operator will talk you through what to do while you wait for an ambulance to arrive.

Trauma care in hospital

There is a growing consensus that major trauma – serious injury where there is a strong possibility of death or disability – is best treated in specialised major trauma centres. Deficiencies in care are common, and there are wide variations in survival: in-hospital mortality rates in the United Kingdom, for example, are 20% higher than in the USA and have barely improved since the 1980s despite repeated calls for action (National Audit Office, 2010). Citing data from the Trauma Audit and Research Network, the National Audit Office blamed substandard care, in which specialised surgical facilities are inadequate, especially at nights and weekends, for poor survival after trauma. These strictures applied with equal force to the variable provision of rehabilitation services across the UK.

The interested reader should consult the many resources and specialist textbooks on first aid, advanced trauma care, regional trauma centres and rehabilitation units.

LEARNING POINT

There is a growing consensus that major trauma – serious injury where there is a strong possibility of death or disability – is best treated in specialised major trauma centres.

SUMMARY OF CHAPTER 8

Combined public health and clinical approaches

Interventions aimed at multiple outcomes

- A distinction may be drawn between preventive interventions that are vertical and those that are horizontal. Vertical interventions are fairly narrowly focused on specific injury types or locations such as roads, schools or homes. Horizontal interventions address the underlying determinants of a range of injuries simultaneously.

- Examples of vertical injury prevention interventions are drink-driver laws and smoke detectors.

- Examples of horizontal injury prevention interventions are safer transport infrastructures (to protect vulnerable pedestrians as well as vehicle occupants), gun control measures (that reduce the incidence of homicide, suicide and unintentional gunshot wounds) and restricting access to potentially harmful medication (thereby reducing the incidence of suicide and unintentional poisoning).

Parenting and early intervention programmes

- Research points to a potentially crucial role for early childhood influences on the later risk of injury. Early intervention studies indicate a range of health, educational and social benefits. And parenting interventions aimed at high-risk families seem to be effective in reducing the incidence of unintentional injuries in children and may promote safer home environments generally.

- A recent systematic review indicates that parenting education and training programmes appear to reduce the risk of injuries in disadvantaged groups, although that does not preclude the possibility that all children might benefit from the interventions.

- Whether these programmes operate through the prevention or amelioration of adverse childhood experiences or as a result of more direct impacts, such as by reducing exposure to environmental hazards and by encouraging the use of safety equipment, is unclear.

Role of clinicians

There are numerous unexploited opportunities for clinicians, including doctors, nurses and other healthcare staff involved in patient care, to become involved in injury prevention. Although routine clinical work may appear to offer limited opportunities for unintentional prevention, there is growing awareness of two principles: prevention and health promotion are core professional responsibilities of all doctors, and that all good clinical management is per se a form of prevention.

With a degree of imagination and initiative, paediatricians and other clinicians can develop and exploit existing clinical services in a way that enables them to contribute more effectively to injury prevention. Examples include:

■ developing injury surveillance in accident and emergency departments, outpatient clinics and inpatient units;

■ identification of children at elevated risk of injury (e.g. repeat attenders, substance misuse);

■ encouraging the implementation or expansion of parenting interventions;

■ offering explicit evidence-based advice and support to parents and carers.

Trauma care – whether in the form of the initial response of emergency services, first aid or subsequent treatment – is a form of tertiary prevention of injury. High-quality intervention by clinicians, emergency teams or even members of the general public can make a difference to an injured person's prognosis. Effective intervention can take place at the scene of the incident, in hospital and following discharge, in the community.

SECTION 3

THE FUTURE

Section 3 Overview

This third and final section looks to the future and identifies some of the key challenges that are likely to face all those around the world who are concerned with injury prevention in the next few decades.

This section comprises four chapters and their summaries:

9. **Changing patterns of health and disease**

10. **Injury prevention in a changing world**

11. **The growing role of knowledge in injury prevention**

12. **Ethical aspects of injury prevention**

CHAPTER 9

Changing patterns of health and disease

Learning objectives

■ To be aware of the pattern of changing global health and injury
■ To have a basic knowledge of the potential impact of globalisation on injury epidemiology
■ To have a basic knowledge of the potential impact of climate change on injury epidemiology
■ To be aware of the way in which changing public health priorities might impact on injury epidemiology

Overview of changing global health

Over the last century or so, there have been major improvements in global health. Death rates have declined, especially in children, and life expectancy has increased. Nevertheless, inequalities in heath between and within regions and countries have remained unchanged or have widened. Health indicators in sub-Saharan Africa, the Middle East and Eastern Europe appear particularly resistant to significant improvement, partly due to the ravages of the HIV/AIDS epidemic and partly through economic stagnation.

The health status of a population reflects the interaction of its genetic make-up and its exposure to a range of environmental influences. Although great advances have been made in genetics in recent decades, such as the mapping of the human genome, most health variation between populations is likely to be due to environmental rather than genetic factors. The implication of this argument is that changing patterns of health are likely to be environmentally rather than generically determined. And a key component of the environment is socio-economic status.

Around a fifth of the world's population live in absolute poverty, while around half have incomes insufficient to meet more than their most basic needs. Although the relationship between wealth and health is complex, poverty remains the single most important underlying determinant of illness and injury in a population. Moreover, income distribution within countries appears to exert an effect on life expectancy: the more economically unequal a country, the lower its average life expectancy (Wilkinson, 1992).

LEARNING POINT

Although the relationship between wealth and health is complex, poverty remains the single most important underlying determinant of illness and injury in a population.

Changing global pattern of injury

Reference has already been made to the World Health Organization Global Burden of Disease Study (see Chapter 2), which has predicted a steadily increasing toll of injury and its consequences across the globe. That may seem surprising given the pattern of decline in injury mortality in most developed countries. Assuming that the developing world follows suit, shouldn't the overall international trend move in a downwards direction?

Crystal ball gazing is always hazardous even when sophisticated epidemiological methods are employed. The term 'horizon scanning' portrays a sense of clarity and certainty that is highly misleading because emerging trends, new threats, changing technologies and novel insights are all hard to decipher in their early stages. Nevertheless, there are several reasons why injuries are likely to become more problematic, in terms of both incidence and severity, for the world in the future:

❑ The 'epidemiological transition' is the process by which countries undergoing rapid economic development experience a shift in the pattern of disease away from nutritional and infectious causes and towards chronic disease, mental illness and injuries. These changes in the pattern of death, sickness and disability, which especially affect younger age groups, are brought about by major shifts in underlying causal factors including demography, behaviour, environment and culture.

❑ The UK and other developed countries underwent this transition around the middle of the 20th century. Many low- and middle-income countries are currently undergoing this and might thus expect to reap its benefits. Unfortunately, this is not necessarily the case. On the contrary, many low-income countries appear to be experiencing the worst of both worlds – a continuing high level of nutritional deficiencies and infections combined with a rapidly increasing burden of chronic disease and injuries.

❑ With increasing industrialisation, car ownership in the developing world tends to increase in response to consumer demand. Although this may yield genuine benefits in terms of increased mobility for a large number of people, it also incurs a cost. As the number of miles driven rises, so does the exposure of pedestrians to vehicles. This inevitably leads to more road casualties of all severities, particularly in vulnerable road users such as children and older people.

❑ As malnutrition, infection and poverty gradually decline in importance, life expectancy increases, consumer demand for and involvement in more

152

hazardous occupational and leisure pursuits (such as driving heavy goods vehicles, the use of sophisticated building equipment and greater participation in sports) reflect this, albeit with some offsetting of this increased risk by the adoption of safer equipment, improvements in road and other environments, and progress in the healthcare and educational sectors.

❑ Economic development generally produces a demographic shift over time towards an older population who add not only to the pool of more vulnerable potential injury victims, incurring greater costs to local and national economies, but also to the number of injury agents (e.g. through driving). The net result will be an increase in the incidence, consequences and costs of injuries.

Whether these trends will continue unabated into the middle of the 21st century is a moot point. The precautionary principle, however, requires us to prepare for the scenario outlined above. There is no place either for complacency or pessimism. By recognising the nature of the threat to our collective future posed by injury, we can respond to it in ways that may avert at least some of its most destructive manifestations.

The impact of globalisation

'Globalisation' is a politicised term that polarises opinion. One view is that it is an inevitable consequence of economic and technological progress and should be recognised as harbouring the potential for both good and ill. Another is that its advocates have a vested interest because it perpetuates the fundamentally exploitative relationship between rich and poor countries. All agree, however, that the phenomenon is real, irreversible and extremely significant.

The health effects of globalisation are undoubtedly both positive and negative, a confusing reality that applies equally to injury. Globalisation may be defined as 'a set of socio-economic, cultural, political and environmental processes that intensify the connections between nations, businesses and people' (Peden *et al.*, 2008, p. 4). The rapid dissemination of information around the world that globalisation promotes is generally beneficial in raising awareness of injury and how to prevent it. On the other hand, the increased movement of goods and people magnifies the risks to which people are exposed either directly, through the marketing of potentially hazardous consumer products, or indirectly, via the expansion of transport and other infrastructures that pose a threat to safety.

◀ LEARNING POINT

The health effects of globalisation are undoubtedly both positive and negative, a confusing reality that applies equally to injury.

Motorisation has probably peaked in most of the developed world, but developing countries cannot progress economically without new roads and vehicles, and these will pose ever-increasing threats to the safety of children.

A related phenomenon is urbanisation, which is also a double-edged sword. Trauma care is more easily organised and delivered in urban than in rural settings, but the proliferation of urban slums creates new and unfamiliar hazards to families and children. This process is therefore likely to lead to substantial increases in both intentional and unintentional injuries in such settings.

Because the world economy is interdependent, an economic crisis in one region has immediate repercussions elsewhere. The international banking crisis of 2008–9 illustrated this reality vividly. Although magnified by a recessionary tendency that was already underway, the collapse of Lehman Brothers, a major US bank, triggered a sequence of events that engulfed all the world's markets, reduced financial liquidity, depressed national economies and prompted massive public expenditure leading to equally vast cuts in services. The effects of these trends on health in general and child safety in particular are unclear but are likely to be negative.

The impact of climate change

Whatever the scientific arguments surrounding its causes, and in particular the role of carbon emissions in producing global warming, climate change is occurring. This will have a negative impact on injury risk and severity. The Intergovernmental Panel on Climate Change (2007) predicts a temperature rise of between 1.5°C and 6°C by 2100 depending on the extent of future emissions. While this remains a wide range, even a small temperature rise will bring about important new challenges to public health, and these will become manifest in various ways in the relatively near future.

●LEARNING POINT

Whatever the scientific arguments surrounding its causes, and in particular the role of carbon emissions in producing global warming, climate change is occurring. This will have a negative impact on injury risk and severity.

As the sea level rises, people will try to migrate in large number from low-lying delta regions to higher ground, and this will generate many hazards. Drowning deaths, in particular, are likely to increase in incidence. Extreme weather conditions – causing floods, typhoons, heatwaves, droughts, desertification and fires – pose direct threats to children's safety. The indirect effects of climate change are less predictable but equally or more worrying from a safety perspective. Among these might be included large and sudden population migrations, economic hardship, civil unrest and interstate conflict over water, oil and other natural resources.

Roberts and Hillman (2009) have pointed out that climate change and injury have energy as a common source. Over 80% of carbon dioxide emissions worldwide are from road transport, and road crashes are responsible for a quarter of all injury mortality. If road transport is reduced in an attempt to control these emissions, injury risk should decline. All the evidence to date, however, suggests that this is an unlikely scenario unless vigorous additional action is taken to propel all countries towards a low-carbon economy. Nevertheless, the imperative to reduce energy use will provide a key policy context for future injury prevention activities.

Changing public health priorities and injury

Although injury per se is not often explicitly mentioned as a public health priority, several other topics currently preoccupying policy-makers have an influence on injury prevention, whether directly or indirectly. Three of these are obesity, social inequalities and the early years.

The correlation between body weight and the risk of injury is unclear. There is a complex relationship between body weight and injury, with both underweight and overweight children at increased risk. What is indisputable, however, is that obesity is widely perceived to pose a major public challenge in almost all countries. Anti-obesity strategies are predicated on two components – reducing caloric intake and increasing exercise. Policies that promote the latter include encouraging children to play, both sports and informally, to cycle, to walk to school and generally to expend more energy both indoors and outdoors. All of these activities are associated with greater exposure to environmental hazards. As obesity is likely to be accorded a higher priority than injury prevention, it is hard to avoid the conclusion that children will be injured in greater numbers as anti-obesity measures are implemented.

◼️ LEARNING POINT

As obesity is likely to be accorded a higher priority than injury prevention, it is hard to avoid the conclusion that children will be injured in greater numbers as anti-obesity measures are implemented.

One of the major failings of public health in the 20th century was its inability to reduce social inequalities in health. Governments around the world have explicitly set inequality reduction as a policy objective, although few appear to have identified convincing solutions to date. As childhood injury mortality is one of the most socially patterned of all health outcomes, a focus on injury prevention will resonate strongly with inequality reduction. This offers a huge opportunity for linking the two agendas in a synergistic way.

The growing early years movement is perhaps the most exciting development in the entire public health landscape. Although the motivation for this may only obliquely relate to injury, with the possible exception of violence prevention, it will have implications for child safety. The early years are viewed, rightly, as holding the key to better behavioural and educational outcomes in childhood, adolescence and early adult life.

A striking example of this was a political pamphlet published by two British Members of Parliament that called for an all-party commitment to early intervention. Their premise was that 'large parts of our society are underachieving and that the financial and social costs of this are both enormous and multiplying' (Allen and Smith, 2008, p. 4). A particularly appealing aspect of this argument to politicians is that the limited econometric data available strongly suggest that substantial savings to the public purse may be achieved through investment in the early years of the life cycle. In their preamble, the MPs wrote:

> We are convinced that it is cheaper and more sensible to tackle problems before they begin rather than spend ever-greater sums on ineffective reme-dial policies, whether they take the form of more prisons, police, drug rehabilitation or supporting longer and more costly lifetimes on benefits.

This clarion call for prevention was endorsed by all the major UK political leaders at the time and provides the most promising vehicle for the creation of a healthier, more successful and safer future for the majority of the world's children.

All of these ideas have a global relevance. The scale, complexity and cost of implementing them effectively requires humankind to work collaboratively. This, in turn, involves adopting an international perspective on the problem. Although the task is daunting, much has already been achieved.

SUMMARY OF CHAPTER 9
Changing patterns of health and disease

- Over the last century or so, there have been major improvements in global health. Death rates have declined, especially in children, and life expectancy has increased. Nevertheless, inequalities in heath between and within regions and countries remain.

- Most health variation between populations is likely to be due to environmental rather than genetic factors. Changing patterns of health are likely to be environmentally rather than generically determined.

- Poverty remains the single most important underlying determinant of illness and injury in a population. Moreover, income distribution within countries appears to exert an effect on life expectancy: the more economically unequal a country, the lower its average life expectancy.

- Injuries are likely to become more problematic, in terms of both incidence and severity, for the world in the future.

- Globalisation is a double-edged sword for injury prevention. For example, motorisation and urbanisation produce both benefits and threats to safety.

- Whatever the scientific arguments surrounding its causes, and in particular the role of carbon emissions in producing global warming, climate change is occurring and has serious implications for injury prevention.

- Perceived public health priorities (obesity, social inequalities and the early years) are changing and will have an impact on injury risk. Children are likely to be injured in greater numbers as anti-obesity measures are implemented.

- A focus on injury prevention will resonate strongly with aspirations to reduce inequality. This offers a huge opportunity for linking the two agendas in a synergistic way.

- The growing early years movement is perhaps the most exciting development in the entire public health landscape. Prevention by this means offers the most promising vehicle for the creation of a healthier, more successful and safer future for the majority of the world's children.

CHAPTER 10

Injury prevention in a changing world

Learning objectives

■ To be aware of the international dimension of injury prevention

■ To have a basic knowledge of the role of international agencies for injury prevention

■ To be aware of the potential role of dedicated injury prevention centres

International dimension – learning from each other

Undertaking international comparisons of injury rates is deeply problematic given the absence of consistent definitions, classification systems and quality standards for such data. Nevertheless, some intriguing patterns are evident. Even after taking account of the vagaries of data collection and reporting, there is undoubtedly a wide variation in injury mortality rates across the globe. There are probably at least three explanations for this. First, mortality partly reflects case fatality and this, in turn, is the outcome of medical care of varying effectiveness. Second, populations are exposed to varying levels of risk arising from social, cultural, economic, political, climactic and geographical factors. Finally, although this is a difficult area to research, it is also likely that varying success in implementing preventive policies and practice in different countries makes a contribution.

Can we identify good child safety practice – ideally best practice – in particular countries? Is there one country above all others that we can look to as a role model for child safety? The answer is probably yes. No country is perfect in this (or any other) regard, but there is a consensus in the injury prevention community that Sweden represents the epitome of good child safety policy and effective implementation. What exactly are the Swedes getting right?

◖LEARNING POINT

Although no country is perfect, a consensus exists in the injury prevention community that Sweden represents the epitome of good child safety policy and effective implementation.

The curious case of Sweden

Is Sweden's strong reputation for child safety justified, or is that country merely the beneficiary of a combination of a helpful historical legacy, a compliant population and a modicum of good luck?

As was described earlier in relation to child maltreatment, Sweden was not always the global star performer. As Hemenway (2009) points out, Swedish children suffered higher injury death rates than American children in the 1950s. Within half a century, however, Swedish rates had slumped to around a third of American rates, and they are now fairly consistently the lowest in the world. The way this was achieved is worth examining in some detail.

The first milestone was the establishment of the Children's Accident Committee in 1954. This comprised voluntary organisations and non-governmental organisations (NGOs) who came together to disseminate a single message – that injury was a public health problem that demanded collective action. The campaign comprised three elements. The first was to create an ambitious system of injury data collection and analysis. The second was to call for a much tighter regulatory framework to promote a safer environment for children whether at home, on the roads or at play. The third was to educate the public relentlessly, using the mass media and other channels, about the avoidability of childhood injuries and the responsibility of parents, teachers and the adult community to protect children from harm. This multifaceted and determined effort, sustained over many years with varying degrees of government support, propelled the country to the top of the international child safety league table.

Bergman and Rivara (1991) identified five factors that contributed to Sweden's success in reducing child injury death rates to such a low level:

- good surveillance data;
- a commitment to research;
- regulation and legislation for safer environments;
- broad based multi-agency safety education campaigns;
- committed leadership on safety issues.

Jansson *et al.* (2006) highlighted four specific factors (some of which overlap with the above):

- the widespread adoption of 'functionalist architecture', with a consequent separation of traffic from pedestrians;
- the expansion of child day care centres;
- the introduction of mandatory swimming lessons for schoolchildren;
- the establishment of local child safety programmes.

Sweden has been in the forefront of countries adopting the recommendations of the World Health Organization (WHO) on safety policy-making and has pioneered the Safe Community concept. As a country, it has a tradition of taking collective responsibility for the welfare of its citizens and has not hesitated to legislate for safety, including stricter consumer product regulations, when necessary. Moreover, academic researchers and campaigning clinicians (such as Dr Ragnar Berfenstam) have been closely involved in national and local policy-making.

Other countries

The only other countries to have challenged Sweden's primacy in child safety are The Netherlands and the UK, both of which have particularly good records on road safety.

As Hemenway (2009) has described, The Netherlands has systematically set about creating an environment that is attractive and safe for pedestrians and cyclists. The country has created physical barriers between traffic and people in residential neighbourhoods, reduced speed limits and established designated recreational zones (*woonerfs*) where pedestrians and cyclists have legal priority over cars. This idea has spread to the UK, Germany, Canada, the USA and elsewhere, although on a very limited scale. The Netherlands has also exploited its flat terrain by building a huge number of cycle paths and ensuring that these are fully integrated into new housing developments. The results have been impressive: both pedestrian and cycling fatalities have fallen by well over half since 1975.

The USA is unquestionably the world leader in injury epidemiological and preventive research. It has taken great strides forward since the publication of *Injury in America* in 1986 and the subsequent financial investment around the country (Christoffel and Gallagher, 2006). The reasons for this success are multiple and complex, but several themes, from which other countries may be able to learn, are discernible.

First, violence and suicide in the USA are now routinely included under the rubric of injury prevention in a way that would have been unheard of a generation ago. Second, there has been a much-expanded research effort aimed at unravelling the causes of injury and developing preventive countermeasures. Third, routine data sources have proliferated, led by the National Center for Health Statistics, which collects many more and detailed data on both injury mortality and morbidity, including mandated external cause coding in several states. Fourth, skills development and capacity building has advanced apace through the National Training Initiative for Injury and Violence Prevention. Fifth, preventive guidelines, good practice manuals, specialist journals and newsletters, many of which are available online, abound. Finally, the close involvement of the Centers for Disease Control, the national public health agency that set up a National Center for Injury Prevention and Control, has been crucial, as has been the formation of nationwide networks such as the Society for the Advancement of Violence and Injury Research and the Safe States Alliance (formerly the State and Territorial Injury Prevention Directors' Association).

In many respects, the USA may be regarded as the world leader in injury research, training, surveillance and control. That country's progress has, however, been severely hampered by its exceptionally high toll of injury mortality and morbidity from firearm injuries.

◼ LEARNING POINT ──────────────────────────

Although the USA may be regarded as the world leader in injury research, training, surveillance and control, its progress has been severely hampered by its exceptionally high toll of injury mortality and morbidity from firearm injuries.

• •

The UK approach to safety has been rather patchy. Its major successes have been in the fields of consumer and road safety. The former may be attributed to a combination of a strong historical tradition of strict regulation of product manufacture and distribution, reinforced by its joining of the European Union with its vigorous framework of standards and enforcement. Government commitment to road safety has always been firm, with the steady application of downwards pressure on road casualty rates via high-quality road engineering, enforcement of safer driving and the use of national casualty reduction targets. A further factor in the UK's reasonably good safety record is the existence of a well-organised voluntary sector, dominated by two NGOs (the Royal Society for the Prevention of Accidents and the Child Accident Prevention Trust) that act (despite receiving a degree of public subsidy) as a powerful and constant reminder to governments of their responsibilities.

Injury prevention in the developing world

Developing countries suffer disproportionately from injuries. More than 95% of child injury deaths worldwide are estimated to occur in low- or middle-income countries. This is partly due to the association of injury with poverty. It may also be attributed to lack of awareness combined with an unwillingness or inability of many governments, faced with many competing priorities, to devote sufficient resources, governmental attention or political impetus to the problem. The scale of the injury problem in poorer countries is difficult to measure due to inadequate data, but there is now overwhelming evidence that every country on earth has become caught up in the global injury pandemic. Economic development has proved a double-edged sword, in injury terms, as it has led to increasing motorisation and urbanisation, both of which have tended to increase the exposure of children to environmental hazards (Peden *et al.*, 2008).

◼ LEARNING POINT ──────────────────────────

More than 95% of all injury deaths in children are estimated to occur in low- or middle-income countries. This is partly due to the association of injury with poverty and partly due to the unwillingness or inability of many governments to devote sufficient resources to the problem.

• •

The response to date has been disappointing overall, although there has been some progress. Child survival programmes, in accordance with the fourth

Millennium Development Goal proclaimed by the United Nations (UN) General Assembly in 2000, have sought to reduce child mortality in the pre-5 age group. The focus has, however, been overwhelmingly on nutritional and infectious diseases, with impressive results in many cases. Millions of lives are believed to have been saved by the implementation of programmes designed to enhance growth monitoring, breastfeeding, immunisation and healthcare. If progress is to be maintained in the future, such programmes must now turn their attention to injury prevention as a matter of urgency.

Role of international agencies

For all their well-publicised faults, the UN and related bodies have generally been a force for good in seeking to highlight the plight of children and their need for protection. Since the Second World War, several UN agencies have played a leading role in international activities. These include the World Bank, the UN Children's Fund (UNICEF), the UN Development Programme and the WHO.

Arguably the most successful (and respected) of these is the WHO. It has achieved the remarkable feat of galvanising global efforts to combat infectious diseases and is widely credited with the eradication of smallpox in the 1970s. In more recent years, the body has suffered from excessive bureaucracy, lack of accountability, distortion of policies through politicisation, uncertain leadership, internal feuding and a perceived decline in effectiveness. Part of the problem has been attributed to an allegedly wide gap between the rhetoric of WHO proclamations such as Health For All by the Year 2000 and its obvious failure to achieve them (Beaglehole and Bonita, 1997).

Five international initiatives are especially worthy of mention in the context of child safety. These are the UN Convention on the Rights of the Child, World Health Assembly Resolutions, the Millennium Development Goals, Child Survival, and the UNICEF Innocenti Report Card.

UN Convention on the Rights of the Child

The UN Convention on the Rights of the Child is a landmark document that has been ratified by most countries. It enshrines three key principles: that children should be provided with essential services to maintain their health and well-being, that children should be protected from hazards in their environment and from exploitation by adults, and that children should participate in decision-making that affects their welfare.

Specifically (in, for example Articles 3, 6, 19, 24, 31 and 32), the Convention asserts that all children have a right to a safe environment and to protection from injury and violence. These requirements apply to the various settings in which children may be found, including the home, care systems, school and employment. In one sense, the Convention is a massive leap forward in the effort to protect children. At the same time, there is no avoiding the fact that these rights are breached on a daily basis in many, if not most, countries. Calling these countries to account, not merely for their failure to adhere to the Convention but also for their hypocrisy in claiming to uphold it, remains a challenge for child safety campaigners around the world.

World Health Assembly Resolutions

The WHA, through its resolutions, has strongly endorsed various reports of the Violence and Injury Prevention and Disability programme (VIP) of the WHO. The VIP has played a major role in raising the international profile of the field by ceaselessly reiterating some key messages: injury being a global (and growing) public health problem; the unequal burden of injury across the globe and between social groups; the preventability of injuries as indicated by research evidence; the multisectoral nature of injury prevention and safety; the need for a comprehensive approach and integration between intentional and unintentional injury prevention programmes; the peculiar vulnerability of children to injury; the legal imperative to protect children enshrined in the Convention on the Rights of the Child; the huge human and financial costs of injury and the potential savings generated by prevention; the continuing inadequacy of existing routine data on injuries at national and local level; and the need for research designed to enhance knowledge about injury causes and prevention.

In their *World Report on Child Injury Prevention*, the WHO (Peden *et al.*, 2008) urged governments and others to take seven actions:

- ❏ to integrate child injury into a comprehensive approach to child health and development;
- ❏ to develop and implement a child injury prevention policy and a plan of action;
- ❏ to implement specific actions to prevent and control child injuries;
- ❏ to strengthen health systems to address child injuries;
- ❏ to enhance the quantity and quality of data for child injury prevention;
- ❏ to define priorities for research, and support research on the causes, consequences, costs and prevention of child injuries;
- ❏ to raise awareness of and target investments towards child injury prevention.

These recommendations were addressed to international development organisations, governments, NGOs, the private sector, the media, teachers and community leaders, parents, and children themselves.

Millennium Development Goals

In 2000, the General Assembly of the UN adopted eight Millennium Development Goals. These have been described as 'the most broadly supported, comprehensive and specific development goals the world has ever agreed upon' (www.undp.org/mdg/basics.shtml accessed 7 February 2011).

The goals relate to poverty, hunger, maternal and child mortality, disease, inadequate shelter, gender inequality, environmental degradation and economic development. They are bound by a time line and address, through concrete numerical benchmarks, strategies to reduce extreme poverty. If these are achieved, world poverty will be halved, millions of lives will be saved and billions of people will benefit from economic progress. The goals are linked to targets and indicators. Progress so far appears to have been mixed: although some inroads have been made into poverty, many of the other targets are likely to be missed. The countries lagging behind are concentrated in especially poor regions of the world, including sub-Saharan Africa and South Asia.

The fourth goal is to reduce, by two-thirds, the mortality rate of children under 5 years between 1990 and 2015. As injuries contribute to around 6% of deaths in the age group 1–4 years, injury prevention efforts will clearly be essential if this goal is to be met.

Child Survival

There are almost 11 million deaths annually in children under the age of 5 years. The Bellagio Study Group on Child Survival, comprising a small number of concerned scientists from around the world, held a series of meetings that also involved the WHO, UNICEF and the World Bank. This culminated in a workshop in Bellagio, Italy, in 2003 sponsored by the Rockefeller Foundation. The Group published an influential series of papers in *The Lancet* in that year that stimulated the 'child survival debate' in various fora. The authors claimed that implementing 23 proven and cost-effective interventions could prevent two-thirds of child deaths (Bellagio Study Group on Child Survival, 2003). To date, much emphasis has been placed upon nutrition, infection and neonatal health; injury prevention has scarcely featured in these discussions, although it clearly deserves greater attention in view of its epidemiological contribution to childhood mortality.

◾LEARNING POINT

In international discussions on child health, much emphasis has been placed upon nutrition, infection and neonatal health. Injury prevention has scarcely featured to date.

UNICEF Innocenti Report Card

In 2001, UNICEF published its Innocenti Report Card No. 2, in which it pointed out that injury had become the leading killer of children aged 1–14 years in every industrialised country, with almost 40% of all deaths in that age group being attributable to this cause. The USA and Portugal had the highest child injury mortality rates and Sweden the lowest. The authors estimated that 12,000 young lives would be saved each year if every rich country had the injury mortality rate of Sweden.

The report found that poverty was correlated with injury mortality rates but in an inconsistent fashion. Other risk factors were single parenthood, low maternal education, low maternal age at birth, poor housing, large family size and parental substance abuse. The authors asserted that much remained to be done to implement preventive measures of proven efficacy. Not one country had legislated in all seven specific areas where safety measures have been shown to work – cycle helmets, speed limits in built-up areas, child safety seats in cars, seat belt wearing in cars by children, child-resistant packaging of medication, smoke detectors in homes and playground safety standards.

Role of dedicated injury prevention centres

The British Medical Association and others have called for a coordinated effort designed to bring together researchers, practitioners and policy-makers concerned with injury prevention. One means of achieving this is to create academic, research or task-oriented 'focal points' or centres. Whatever approach is adopted, the experience of other countries suggests (e.g. New Zealand, Australia, the USA and Sweden) that there is a clear need to avoid fragmentation, to achieve a critical mass of expertise and to encourage a multidisciplinary approach to the complex issues surrounding injury and safety. This has led to the creation of dedicated injury prevention centres, often funded by national regional governments, to take forward this agenda. These centres seem to work best when they are content not just to generate purely 'academic' output, but rather to combine this with an action-oriented programme of advocacy, training and campaigning. Sceptics point to the set-up and running costs of such centres and to the lack of evidence that such organisations contribute more to injury prevention than the alternative and allegedly less effective fragmented approach that is pursued in most countries.

SUMMARY OF CHAPTER 10

Injury prevention in a changing world

- Even after taking account of the vagaries of data collection and reporting, there is undoubtedly a wide variation in injury mortality rates across the globe.

- There is a consensus in the injury prevention community that Sweden represents the epitome of good child safety policy and effective implementation.

- Developing countries suffer disproportionately from injuries. More than 95% of all injury deaths in children are estimated to occur in low- or middle-income countries.

- For all their well-publicised faults, the United Nations and related bodies (especially the World Health Organization) have generally been a force for good in seeking to highlight the plight of children and their need for protection.

- There is a clear need to avoid fragmentation, to achieve a critical mass of expertise and to encourage a multidisciplinary approach to the complex issues surrounding injury and safety. This has led to the creation of dedicated injury prevention centres, often funded by national regional governments.

CHAPTER 11

The growing role of knowledge in injury prevention

Learning objectives

■ To be aware of the expanding research effort on injury prevention

■ To understand the importance of awareness-raising, dissemination of evidence and closing the knowledge–practice implementation gap

■ To understand the importance and limitations of educating the public in injury prevention

■ To have an awareness of the key role of professional education in injury prevention

■ To be aware of recent advances in violence prevention research

The expanding research effort

Our understanding of the epidemiology, causes, consequences and prevention of injuries is almost entirely dependent on knowledge generated by high-quality scientific research. A frequently articulated complaint from injury prevention practitioners and policy-makers is that the evidence base is too weak due to the scarcity of research studies and publications. This may well have been true in the past and probably reflected a lack of funding for injury research. In the UK, for example, the Department of Health funded a strategic review of research priorities for unintentional injury in 1999 (Ward and Christie, 2000) that highlighted the gross under-funding of injury research and called for a comprehensive, collaborative approach to injury prevention research. More recent data from the UK Clinical Research Collaboration, quoted by Nicholl (2006), showed that injury contributes 6.6% of UK disability-adjusted life–years yet received only 0.3% of health research funding in 2004–5 – a 22-fold discrepancy.

Nevertheless, it is instructive to observe the striking upsurge in the number of publications in the field in the last two decades. Stone (1996) complained that the research community had been slow to respond to the challenge posed by injuries, partly due to an inherent resistance on the part of many national agencies to allocating resources to this type of investigation. Other obstacles included the lack of international consensus around definitions, and classification and coding systems, a deficiency being addressed by the International Collaborative Effort on Injury Statistics of the National Institutes of Health (Fingerhut, 2004). Stone (1996) proposed that an international research agenda be drawn up in accordance with a single overarching criterion – meeting the needs of injury prevention. He summarised those needs as threefold:

- ❑ to understand the epidemiology and natural history of injuries;
- ❑ to select appropriate preventive interventions;
- ❑ to evaluate the impact of these interventions.

Pless (2006) charted the history of peer review publications worldwide using the search terms 'injury prevention' or 'accident prevention' and noted an increase from one paper in 1946 to nearly 2000 by 2005. Although he questioned whether this massive expansion in research was having an impact on injury rates, he nevertheless celebrated the undoubted numerical trend as an encouraging sign of progress.

Quantity does not necessarily equate to quality, of course, and these numbers are a relatively crude means of documenting research output. Furthermore, whether this rapidly proliferating body of knowledge is perceived as relevant to supporting evidence-based injury prevention policy and practice is another matter entirely. Yet it seems we have entered a relatively information-rich era of injury prevention, and that bodes well for the future.

Villavecas et al. (2010) proposed a common set of principles that could form the basis of a global injury prevention research agenda. These included:

- ❑ agreeing on terminology and definitions;
- ❑ recognising the need for multiple disciplinary perspectives;
- ❑ building capacity through training, translation, implementation and dissemination;
- ❑ promoting partnership working between government departments, communities and academic centres;
- ❑ addressing mass injury events, whether natural or human-made.

Awareness-raising, dissemination of evidence and closing the knowledge-practice implementation gap

This book, and others like it, argues that injury is an important and avoidable source of human death, disability and suffering in the 21st century. However, this key message has yet to permeate the consciousness of the public, professionals and politicians. One stumbling block is the way injury is reported in routine statistics. The thoughtful and detailed analysis of Wanless (2004), for example, entirely missed (in his initial tabulation) the pre-eminent position of injury in the premature mortality league table for England (Table 11.1), probably because of the fragmentation of injury causes into subcategories (road casualties, suicide, etc.). By simply adding together the various injury causes, and assuming that 1% of the 'other causes' are in related to injury, injury leaps to the top of the table (Table 11.2).

Top Causes (%) Of Years Of Life Lost To Age 75, England 1999

CHD	18
Cancer	17
Injury/poisoning	*9*
Suicide/undetermined	*6*
Stroke	6
Respiratory disease	6
Liver disease (alcohol related)	2
Road traffic accidents	*2*
Diabetes	1
Others	33
TOTAL	100

Source: Wanless Report 2003

Table 11.1 Wanless Report – original table. CHD, coronary heart disease. The italics indicate injury causes.

Top Causes (%) of Years of Life Lost to Age 75, England 1999 (Revised Version)

Injury/poisoning/suicide/RTAs	*18*
CHD	18
Cancer	17
Stroke	6
Respiratory disease	6
Liver disease (alcohol related)	2
Diabetes	1
Others	32
TOTAL	100

Source: Wanless Report 2003

Table 11.2 Wanless Report – table revised by current author. CHD, coronary heart disease; RTA, road traffic accident. The italics indicate injury causes.

Much is already being done to prevent injury, so what is the scope for further action? Declining injury mortality may reflect improving case-fatality rates in victims due to better quality trauma care (Roberts *et al.*, 1996) rather than declining incidence. A reasonable assumption is that a cluster of countermeasures – such as car seat belts, drink-driving laws, child-resistant containers and fire-proof nightwear – have contributed to the observed fall in injury mortality, but the empirical data are inadequate to draw firm conclusions. Other possible explanations for declining child injury mortality include reduced exposure to hazards (e.g. children being taken by car to school rather than walking), and changing recording and classification practices (e.g. an increasing recognition of other causes of death such as child abuse or adverse effects of medical care).

Much existing knowledge based on high-quality research about what works in injury prevention has indeed found its way into policy, but a wide implementation gap remains even in the world's wealthiest countries (Towner and Towner, 2001). Examples of the failure to apply such knowledge in the UK and elsewhere include the haphazard enforcement of speed limits, the limited deployment of speed cameras or radar traps, the continued marketing of baby walkers, the absence of legislation to ensure the wearing of cycle helmets, the non-use of daytime running lights on cars and the persistent toleration of physical methods of punishing children.

LEARNING POINT

Much existing knowledge based on high-quality research about what works in injury prevention has found its way into policy, but a wide implementation gap remains even in the world's wealthiest countries.

Rivara and Grossman (1996), while commending the efforts of the US public health community (including the National Center for Injury Prevention and Control that had been set up within the Centers for Disease Control and Prevention), argued strongly against complacency in the light of declining unintentional injury mortality rates. They estimated that a further 31% (6,640 per year) of child injury deaths could be avoided in the USA by the full implementation of injury prevention measures of known efficacy.

There have been few studies in other countries, but it seems likely that these US estimates could apply across the globe and may even be quite conservative. Petridou et al. (2007) attempted to quantify the potential for saving lives in 25 European Union (EU) countries if all countries experienced the same unintentional mortality rates in children (0–14 years) as the country with the lowest rate (Sweden). They concluded that nearly half of deaths might be avoidable, while acknowledging the numerous pitfalls in offering such speculation. Geographical differences could reflect methodological variation in data collection, analysis and reporting, lifestyle or risk factors that impinge on injury, as well as (or instead of) the impact of specific preventive measures. A similar study (Stone et al., 2006) suggested that over two-thirds of homicide and suicide deaths in children might have been avoided each year in the EU if all countries had matched the rate reported by the country (Greece) reporting the lowest rates. Again, the extent to which this theoretical figure could actually be achieved is unclear.

In both of these studies, the dependence on mortality data raises the possibility that some of the international variation could be due to the availability and effectiveness of trauma care facilities rather than to either varying risk factor prevalence or the implementation of preventive practices.

Educating the public

The phenomenal growth of the Internet has created unprecedented opportunities for the general public to access quickly and easily numerous authoritative sources of information on health, healthcare and other services. Some of this information is undoubtedly extremely valuable and conducive to health, well-being and safety. Unfortunately, its very accessibility is a double-edged sword since the content of the Internet is less subject to quality control than are more conventional sources of information such as magazines or books.

In the safety field, there are outstanding examples of high-quality resources on safety promotion, some of which have been cited earlier in the book (e.g. first aid advice). In the UK, two notably respected sources are the Child Accident Prevention Trust (CAPT; Shttp://capt.org.uk accessed 7 February 2011) and the Royal Society for the Prevention of Accidents (RoSPA; www.rospa.com/default.aspx accessed 7 February 2011). These non-governmental organisations offer a wide range of information to parents, children, professionals and the wider public in the form of briefing notes, safety advice, quizzes, leaflets, booklets and posters, and weblinks. Some of this information is free of charge.

A key annual educational event in the CAPT calendar is Child Safety Week, in which local child safety groups are encouraged to raise awareness in their localities of the risks posed to children by environmental and other hazards. Described by CAPT as its 'flagship community education campaign', Child Safety Week is aimed at anyone working with families and children. In 2009, it was estimated, through independent polling, to have reached six million people through thousands of local activities. Its philosophy is to try to empower families to take action to enhance safety rather than to tell them what to do.

RoSPA has an all-age remit but contains advice on child safety, whether at home, on the roads or at play. Two notable features of their work are Safety and Risk Education (mainly aimed at schools) and an ambitious home safety equipment loan scheme that they implement with UK government sponsorship. This is aimed particularly at disadvantaged families in areas with the highest child injury rates. It was launched following the publication of an Audit Commission/Healthcare Commission (2007) report that was highly critical of government for its inadequate response to the challenge of childhood injury.

From health education of the public to professional education

Public health agencies around the world have long abandoned the archaic notion that health education could hold the key to health improvement – although sectors of the media and some politicians remain strongly wedded to the idea. Nevertheless, the disappointing impact of exclusively behavioural or educationally based measures on injury incidence should not divert attention from the need to apply education in a different context, namely that of professionals and policy-makers working in the field. Capacity-building through knowledge and skills development of the workforce is one of the cornerstones of a comprehensive approach to injury prevention.

◄ LEARNING POINT ►━━━━━━━━━━━━━━━━━━━━━━━━━━━

Capacity-building through knowledge and skills development of the workforce is one of the cornerstones of a comprehensive approach to injury prevention.
• •

The World Health Organization (WHO) has developed, in conjunction with a network of injury prevention experts, a pioneering and freely available educational programme called TEACH-VIP (www.who.int/violence_injury_prevention/capacitybuilding/teach_vip/en/ accessed 7 February 2011).

A survey of 82 medical schools in 31 countries undertaken in 2002–3 revealed that 60% of schools did not cover basic injury prevention concepts while placing considerable emphasis on treatment and emergency care (Villaveces et al., 2005). The postgraduate medical education scene is equally devoid of injury prevention courses in most countries. In the UK, a postgraduate course on child injury prevention ran for a number of years at the University of Newcastle, with the support of the Department of Health and the CAPT, but proved extremely difficult to sustain.

In the USA, a remarkable educational initiative has been launched jointly by the Safe States Alliance (formerly the State and Territorial Injury Prevention Directors Association) and the Society for the Advancement of Violence and Injury Research (SAVIR). They have developed a set of nine Core Competencies in injury and/or violence prevention (Box 11.1) along with detailed learning objectives. Its purpose is to describe a common understanding of the essential skills and knowledge necessary to work in the field of injury prevention. Its target audience is multidisciplinary, spanning fields such as public health, law enforcement, emergency medical services, occupational health and safety, road and traffic safety, and education. An accompanying text (Thygerson *et al.*, 2008) elaborates these ideas within this educational framework. It remains to be seen whether this highly structured approach to professional skills development will prove sustainable in the USA and be exportable to other countries.

Box 11.1 The USA National Training Initiative of STIPDA and SAVIR:

The Core Competencies for Injury and Violence Prevention

1. Ability to describe and explain injury and/or violence as a major social and health problem.

2. Ability to access, interpret, use and present injury and/or violence data.

3. Ability to design and implement injury and/or violence prevention activities.

4. Ability to evaluate injury and/or violence prevention activities.

5. Ability to build and manage an injury and/or violence prevention program.

6. Ability to disseminate information related to injury and/or violence prevention to the community, other professionals, key policy makers and leaders through diverse communication networks.

7. **Ability to stimulate change related to injury and/or violence prevention through policy, enforcement, advocacy, and education.**

8. **Ability to maintain and further develop competency as an injury and/or violence prevention professional.**

9. **Demonstrate the knowledge, skills, and best practices necessary to address at least one specific injury and/or violence topic (e.g. motor vehicle occupant injury, intimate partner violence, fire and burns, suicide, drowning, child injury, etc.) and be able to serve as a resource regarding that area.**

Source: http://safestates.org/associations/5805/files/Core%20Competencies.pdf (accessed 7 February 2011).

Violence research

Until recently, most violence research addressed downstream manifestations of violent behaviour and how it could be modified through either the criminal justice or the healthcare (mainly psychiatric) system. Generalisable knowledge rarely emerged, partly because of the lack of reliable basic epidemiological data. A UK report, for example, highlighted the small proportion (12%) of the worst cases of sexual violence being reported to the police and the wholly inadequate knowledge about the extent of child maltreatment (McVeigh *et al.*, 2005). The disappointing findings from traditional approaches led, slowly but surely, towards the exploration of research questions relating to causation and prevention. To date, the results are mixed but harbour great promise.

The UK WAVE Trust (Hosking and Walsh, 2005) has repeatedly urged governments and local authorities to implement existing knowledge on violence prevention. It has advocated a coordinated research response involving the large-scale implementation and evaluation of separate or combined interventions directed at the early years. The role of dysfunctional parenting, in which empathy and attunement with infants is absent or inadequate, is now well established as a key aetiological factor for subsequent failings in development, health and the capacity to form and sustain relationships – all of which increase the risk of the individual becoming either a victim or a perpetrator of violence in later life. Moreover, more extreme forms of early exposure are very closely correlated with a propensity to later aggression, antisocial behaviour and violence. The infant brain is hypersensitive to the stress hormones that are secreted in response to adverse experiences such as abuse, and this is the window of opportunity for both protective interventions and the nurturing of parenting skills in future generations. The Trust argues that this knowledge base is now robust enough on act as a base for action combined with careful evaluation.

◄ LEARNING POINT ━━━━━━━━━━━━━━━━━━━━━━━━━━━━━━

The infant brain is hypersensitive to the stress hormones that are secreted in response to adverse experiences such as abuse, and this is the window of opportunity for both protective interventions and the nurturing of parenting skills in future generations.
• •

This proposal is a variant of the WHO view that a public health approach to violence is necessary. The four key steps have a strong research flavour reflecting the fact that public health interventions are (or should be) inevitably closely linked both to the evidence based and to ongoing evaluation. The four steps are as follows:

1. Identify as much knowledge on violence as possible through the systematic collection of data on the extent, type, characteristics and consequences of violence.

2. Research why violence occurs, the risk factors for involvement in violence, and which factors can be change to reduce violence.

3. Explore what works to prevent violence, through the implementation, monitoring and evaluation of interventions.

4. Implement successful interventions in a range of settings, widely disseminating information and establishing cost-effectiveness.

SUMMARY OF CHAPTER 11

The growing role of knowledge in injury prevention

■ Much existing knowledge based on high-quality research about what works in injury prevention has indeed found its way into policy, but a wide implementation gap remains even in the world's wealthiest countries.

■ Examples of the failure to apply knowledge include the haphazard enforcement of speed limits, the limited deployment of speed cameras or radar traps, the continued marketing of baby walkers, the absence of legislation to ensure the wearing of cycle helmets, the non-use of daytime running lights on cars, and the persistent toleration of physical methods of punishing children.

■ The phenomenal growth of the Internet has created unprecedented opportunities for the general public to access quickly and easily numerous authoritative sources of information on health, healthcare and other services.

■ Some of the newly accessible information is undoubtedly extremely valuable and conducive to health, well-being and safety. Unfortunately, its very accessibility is a double-edged sword since the content of the Internet is less subject to quality control than are more conventional sources of information such as magazines or books.

■ The disappointing impact of exclusively behavioural or educationally based measures on injury incidence should not divert attention from the need to apply education in a different context, namely that of professionals and policy-makers working in the field.

■ Capacity-building through knowledge and skills development of the workforce is one of the cornerstones of a comprehensive approach to injury prevention. Education for both undergraduates and postgraduates in the healthcare field is notable by its absence, although there is a small number of new initiatives that show promise.

CHAPTER 12

Ethical aspects of injury prevention

Learning objectives

■ To have a basic knowledge of the ethical principles of healthcare and public health practice
■ To be aware of the ethical aspects of injury prevention
■ To be able to describe some of the ethical conflicts in injury prevention

Ethics of public health practice

The relationship between the general public and the healthcare (and related) professions is often said to be built on trust. Preserving that trust depends, in turn, on professionals' ability to demonstrate to the public a commitment to high standards of competence and behaviour. Professionals demonstrate this commitment via their adherence to moral principles that are either implicit or explicitly enshrined in codes of professional practice. These codes are promulgated and upheld by professional bodies such as the UK General Medical Council and the medical Royal Colleges (including the multidisciplinary Faculty of Public Health).

Ethics, in this context, thus refers to the rules or standards governing the conduct of a person or the members of a profession. Those standards are underpinned by implicit or explicit moral values. Gillon (1994), drawing on the work of American ethicists, argued that healthcare workers should be guided by four fundamental prima facie moral principles:

- ☐ autonomy (respect for individual rights);
- ☐ beneficence (doing good);
- ☐ non-maleficence (avoiding doing harm);
- ☐ justice (ensuring fairness);

as well as a concern for the scope of their application (i.e. to whom or to what do these moral principles apply?).

These four principles, while attracting some criticism, have won broad acceptance among clinicians as they are simple, accessible and culturally neutral. They are also comprehensible to an intelligent lay observer. Yet they may encounter problems when they are applied, in unmodified form, to public health.

A concern for ethics that is relevant specifically to public health has arisen relatively recently and is often framed in terms that imply a need to extend traditional bioethics from individuals to populations. Initially, much attention was paid to the need to consider Gillon's four principles in relation to large numbers of individuals ('a population') in a manner that did not differ fundamentally from the approach of clinicians. In other words, while the scope of application of the principles was larger in scale in the case of public health than in that of clinical practice, the principles themselves were largely identical. That ethical perspective, while superficially appealing, is now recognised as inadequate.

Just as public health is not merely clinical medicine on a large scale, so the ethical aspects of public health are not merely the ethics of clinical medicine applied to populations. While clinical medicine and related fields have developed ethical codes that relate to the appropriate interaction between professionals and individuals in ways that fulfil the four key moral principles described by Gillon, public health workers have to grapple with an entirely different – or at least more complex – set of principles (Kass, 2004). These include advocacy for a fair distribution of resources and the aspiration towards a more socially just society. Both of these involve a consideration of the role of collective responsibilities, commitments and actions to promote and protect the health and safety of communities. There may even, on occasions, arise conflicts between the rights of communities to be protected from health hazards on the one hand, and those of individuals to pursue their own chosen lifestyles on the other. To complicate matters further, the peculiar ethical conundrums posed by the healthcare of young children become even more challenging when scaled up to child public health practice and policy-making.

◀ LEARNING POINT

Just as public health is not merely clinical medicine on a large scale, so the ethical aspects of public health are not merely the ethics of clinical medicine applied to populations.

Ethics of injury prevention

Injury prevention, like all areas of public health practice, is not value-free. It contains at least three implicit moral values or positions.

First, the decision to prevent injury requires a posture of presumed beneficence that is predicated on the assumption that the intervention will actually work or will at least generate a net benefit to society. Since most prevention has a cost, in terms of either resources or undesirable side effects, it may be necessary to adopt a utilitarian perspective that weighs the costs and benefits.

Second, the two most effective strategic approaches to injury prevention (environmental modification and enforcement of legislation) imply a major role for the state or government agencies that some people with a libertarian world view may find philosophically or politically problematic, a discomfort reflected in media portrayals of the 'nanny state'.

Third, the allocation of resources to injury prevention usually involves the denial of those resources to other deserving causes. Distinguishing between competing demands is often controversial, and the final decision may be difficult to justify, even if investing in safety is known to reap long-term net benefits and cost savings.

The above discussion has focused on injury prevention as a 'higher level' public health activity and on the ethical aspects of working with populations rather than individuals. Across the gamut of injury prevention activities, however, there are often more immediate ethical obligations on practitioners who work in explicitly clinical settings (e.g. public health nurses and emergency department staff) to which the traditional healthcare ethical code clearly applies. The specific ethical obligations associated with one particularly challenging form of 'clinical' intervention – screening for disorders or risk factors – were described in Chapter 4.

◀━LEARNING POINT━━━━━━━━━━━━━━━━━━━━━━━━━

The two most effective strategic approaches (environmental modification and enforcement of legislation) imply a major role for the state or government agencies that some people may find philosophically or politically problematic.
● ●

Resolving ethical conflicts in injury prevention

Public health policy may incorporate competing and conflicting values. At the heart of ethical concerns about injury prevention lies a potential clash of values between the state and its citizens, or between public health agencies and individuals. Some preventive measures – such as legislation to outlaw drink-driving or the removal of an abused child to a place of safety – may infringe personal autonomy. Others – such as traffic calming by means of speed bumps – may impair efficient service delivery.

It may seem obvious that ensuring the safety of a population is a supreme social objective to which no sane person would object. But that is not the case. We have seen how divisive is the concept of a 'just war'. That may seem an extreme example, yet obtaining a universal consensus around safety promotion may be equally challenging. In popular culture in the UK, for example, the term 'health and safety' has acquired a pejorative flavour to the point where it is regularly cited by satirists and comedians as epitomising the absurdity of much government interference in everyday life. Indeed, Wikler (quoted by Kass, 2004, p. 233) has argued: 'It is not self-evident that this vision of a safe society, with its lack of immoderation, stress, and risk-taking, is to be favoured over others whose constitutive elements have incidental adverse effects upon health'. In 2010, for instance, the newly elected UK government signalled that it would no longer offer unqualified support for speed cameras as a method of traffic calming – despite the strong evidence of their effectiveness in reducing injury incidence – if local authorities, responding to driver opinion, decided to adopt alternative approaches.

◄ LEARNING POINT ▶───────────────────────

It may seem obvious that ensuring the safety of a population is a supreme social objective to which no sane person would object. But that is not the case.
● ●

Because social justice is so closely correlated with good health – including lower injury rates – injury prevention practitioners and policy-makers may feel impelled to strive for a reduction in poverty and a reduction in social inequalities. Although there is some evidence that such actions can achieve health benefits, a direct dose–response relationship between social inequality reduction and reductions in injury incidence has yet to be convincingly demonstrated. Moreover, the implementation of policies designed to reduce social inequalities by public health professionals could be defined as an overtly 'political' objective that has the potential, at least, to generate conflict with colleagues, politicians and even large swathes of the general public.

Child injury prevention can generate particular tensions between methodological, ideological or attitudinal polarities – populations versus individuals, prevention versus cure, unintentional versus intentional injury, young versus old. And the adoption of an evidence-based approach, with its emphasis on data-driven policy and practice, and a prominent role for evaluation ('to determine the value of') can hardly be regarded as value-free. At the very least, practitioners have to take account of data confidentiality and protection, and the ability or otherwise of people to consent to participate in activities relating to information collection (e.g. injury surveillance), preventive intervention (e.g. screening) or research.

Resolving conflicting ethical imperatives can be as fraught within injury prevention as in every other branch of healthcare and public health. By learning from the experience of those who have grappled with analogous dilemmas in other fields, injury prevention policy-makers and practitioners can find a way forward. Without being overly prescriptive, a good starting point might be to try to adhere as closely as possible to some principles of ethical injury prevention. These might include the articulation of the moral or ethical framework (e.g. the Gillon principles or utilitarianism) within which they are operating, estimating, where feasible, the balance of costs and benefits between the competing options, citing the evidence base, including its strengths and weaknesses, on which the decision-making is dependent, and adopting an open and transparent decision-making process that is open to challenge, debate and review.

◖PRACTICE NUGGET◗

In striving for **ethical injury prevention**, try to adhere to explicit principles whereby the practitioner or policy-maker strives:

- to articulate the moral or ethical framework (e.g. the Gillon principles, utilitarianism) within which they are operating;

- to estimate, where feasible, the balance of costs and benefits between the competing options;

- to cite the evidence base, including its strengths and weaknesses, on which the decision-making is dependent;

- to adopt an open and transparent decision-making process that is open to challenge, debate and review.

Public health is unusual in the context of medical practice in that it has been granted, in most countries, statutory authority to protect the health of the population. There is a widespread recognition that public health cannot be viewed exclusively through the prism of a bioethical tradition that has evolved in response to the perceived need to take account of the welfare and rights of individuals. Nevertheless, populations are composed of individuals, and it would be unreasonable to exempt either public health generally or injury prevention specifically from rigorous and systematic ethical scrutiny.

◖LEARNING POINT◗

It would be unreasonable to exempt either public health generally or injury prevention specifically from rigorous and systematic ethical scrutiny.

SUMMARY OF CHAPTER 12

Ethical aspects of injury prevention

- The decision to prevent injury requires a posture of presumed beneficence that is predicated on the assumption that the intervention will actually work. Since most prevention has a cost, in terms of either resources or undesirable side effects, it may be necessary to adopt a utilitarian perspective.

- Some countermeasures – such as legislation to outlaw drink-driving or the removal of an abused child to a place of safety – may infringe personal autonomy. Others – such as traffic calming by means of speed bumps – may impair efficient service delivery.

- The two most effective strategic approaches (environmental modification and enforcement of legislation) imply a major role for government that some people may find philosophically or politically problematic, a discomfort reflected in media portrayals of the 'nanny state'.

- The allocation of resources to injury prevention usually involves the denial of those resources to other deserving causes, and distinguishing between them may be difficult to justify, even if investing in safety is known to reap long-term benefits and cost savings.

- Public health policy may incorporate competing and conflicting values. Child injury prevention can generate tensions between methodological, ideological or attitudinal polarities – populations versus individuals, prevention versus cure, unintentional versus intentional injury, young versus old.

- Injury prevention practitioners and policy-makers may feel impelled to strive for a reduction in economic poverty and a reduction in social inequalities. This has the potential, at least, to generate tensions with colleagues, politicians and large swathes of the general public.

- The adoption of an evidence-based approach, with its emphasis on data-driven policy and practice, and a prominent role for evaluation ('to determine the value of') can hardly be regarded as value-free. At the very least, practitioners have to take account of data confidentiality and protection, and the ability or otherwise of people to consent to participate.

- It would be unreasonable to exempt either public health generally or injury prevention specifically from rigorous and systematic ethical scrutiny.

Key messages of the book

Chapter 1. Introduction, concepts, definitions, history

- Injuries and violence are threats to health in every country and every community.
- Injury has only recently come to be perceived as a public health problem that merits sustained attention.
- Injuries are not random events but are predictable and avoidable.
- The term 'accident' is becoming obsolete in the professional literature.
- The dichotomy between unintentional and intentional injury is increasingly regarded as untenable.
- Although injury prevention has ancient origins, the writings of Haddon in the 20th century laid the foundations for its modern development.

Chapter 2. Epidemiology and natural history of injury

- The public health importance of injury derives from its epidemiology.
- Declining injury mortality may reflect diminishing exposure, improved trauma care or increased survival rather than declining incidence.
- Injury-related mortality is expected to rise up the Global Burden of Disease league table.
- Injury mortality and hospitalisation rates are liable to contain numerous sources of error.
- Large numbers of injuries present to health services in ways that are not captured by routine statistics.
- Because injury is such a universal human experience, we need to distinguish between injury that is significant from a preventive perspective and injury that is not.
- International variations in injury mortality are striking and difficult to interpret.
- While boys are generally at higher risk of injury than girls, the gender difference in injury risk is non-existent in neonates and increases with age.
- Injury is one of the most strongly socially patterned of disorders.
- Injury risk is, to a large extent, developmentally determined.
- Unintentional injuries form the bulk of all injuries in most populations.
- Most intentional injuries are self-inflicted rather than due to assault.
- The prevalence of deliberate self-harm is hard to determine but could be as high as one in 10 young people aged 11–25 years.
- Violence, like injury as a whole, is becoming recognised as a public health challenge that causes death, injury, disability and suffering to large numbers of people.

181

- The onset of physical aggression occurs in early childhood and steadily declines in most children.
- Empathy is probably is the greatest single inhibitor of the propensity to violence.
- Group violence continues to take a heavy toll of lives and suffering around the world.
- Mental health has a role in the aetiology of most types of injury.

Chapter 3. Preventive approaches to injury

- The public health approach to any problem is analogous to the clinical triad of diagnosis, treatment and follow-up.
- A specialised and extremely popular form of 'community diagnosis' in the injury prevention field is surveillance.
- The second step in the public health approach requires a distillation of the research evidence to identify efficacious interventions.
- The third public health step demands an evaluation, audit or monitoring mechanism to determine the strengths and weaknesses of current interventions.
- It is likely that at least a third of all childhood injury deaths could be avoided were interventions of known efficacy implemented.
- Two of the most popular conceptual models of injury prevention are the three levels (primary, secondary and tertiary) of prevention and the three Es (education, enforcement and engineering/environment).
- Injury prevention should represent an outstanding financial investment.
- Health ministries should take the lead in injury prevention as injury is first and foremost a public health challenge.

Chapter 4. Implementation and evaluation

- Injury prevention policy-making at national level or regional level is a highly complex process.
- Evaluation is easier to support in principle than to perform in practice.
- Evaluation undertaken in the context of research is useful in yielding information about what can work (efficacy); this kind of evaluation is sometimes distinguished from investigations that assess what does work (effectiveness).
- The gold standard method for generating evidence arising from evaluation is the meta-analysis or systematic review of randomised controlled trials.
- Evaluation is often constructed theoretically in relation to objectives across the three dimensions of structure–process–outcome (or sometimes 'impact').
- Screening should be subjected to a specialised form of evaluation because of the unique ethical concerns relating to it.
- Absence of evidence of efficacy is not the same as evidence of absence of efficacy.

Chapter 5. From theory to practice

- All injury prevention begins with a rather abstract idea or vision that then evolves, often in fits and starts, into a plan, strategy, policy, programme or initiative.

- An evidence-based approach does not mean that the practitioner is required to suspend professional judgement.
- The three components of an evidence-based approach – assessing the evidence, professional judgement and involving the public – are equally important.
- Not all preventive measures need to be based on knowledge derived from randomised controlled trials.
- In the past, there was a common and mistaken belief that large sections of the general public, particularly in disadvantaged communities, were either unaware of or uninformed about safety matters.
- Empirical research demonstrates that people are acutely aware of the dangers posed to their children but may feel powerless to take the necessary preventive action.
- Children and young people worry about being injured, although they may think they already know enough to stay safe.

Chapter 6. Implementing unintentional injury prevention
What works in unintentional child injury prevention?
Interventions that reduce injury incidence, severity or risk – roads
- Apply area-wide urban safety measures.
- Promote average traffic speed reduction in both residential and rural areas.
- Improve the enforcement of seat belt/child restraint legislation.
- Encourage the universal wearing of bicycle or motorcycle helmets.
- Facilitate modifications to vehicle design.
- Implement community-based education/advocacy measures to protect pedestrians.

Interventions that reduce injury incidence, severity or risk – homes
- Promote the use of child-resistant closures and packaging.
- Provide, distribute, install and maintain smoke detectors/alarms/sprinklers.
- Ensure a safe temperature of domestic hot water via thermostatic mixing valves.
- Install window safety mechanisms to prevent falls from heights.
- Encourage the installation of stair gates at the tops of stairs.
- Implement parenting support/early intervention home visiting programmes.
- Seek to eliminate or modify baby walkers.
- Seek to eliminate or modify cigarette lighters and cigarettes (self-extinguishing).
- Promote the sale and wearing of non-flamable sleepwear.

Interventions that reduce injury incidence, severity or risk – elsewhere
- Promote the use of personal flotation devices for water recreation.
- Increase the presence of adequately trained lifeguards at water recreational facilities.
- Seek the implementation of isolation fencing around private swimming pools.
- Construct energy-absorbent surfaces in playgrounds.
- Install playground equipment of an appropriate height (1.5 m for young children).

(8 of 27)

Infrastructure interventions that promote safety

- Develop comprehensive population-wide safety strategies and implementation plans.
- Identify strong leadership for developing vision, direction and integration.
- Improve the collection, dissemination and use of national, regional and local injury data.
- Create a focal point to plan, implement and evaluate safety measures.
- Enhance the capacity of and infrastructure for injury prevention.
- Allocate resources for undertaking research, development, monitoring and evaluation.

Chapter 7. Implementing intentional injury prevention

- The only interventions that have clearly been shown to be effective in reducing suicide and deliberate self-harm rates in younger age groups are school-based interventions aimed at adolescents, physician education in suicide recognition and treatment, and restriction of access to lethal suicide means.
- Primary preventive approaches to deliberate self-harm include early interventions such as parenting support and the nurturing of emotionally healthy school environments.
- The public health approach to interpersonal violence requires a paradigm shift from viewing it as a consequence of 'criminal behaviour' in individuals towards overlapping 'pathological processes' at individual, relationship, community and societal levels.
- To undertake primary violence prevention, early (0–3 years of age) intervention could hold the key.
- A multi-pronged approach is necessary to reduce the incidence of collective violence.

Chapter 8. Combined public health and clinical approaches

- A distinction may be drawn between preventive interventions that are vertical and those that are horizontal.
- Research points to a potentially crucial role for early childhood influences on the later risk of injury.
- Parenting education and training programmes appear to reduce the risk of injuries in disadvantaged groups, although that does not preclude the possibility that all children might benefit from the interventions.
- There are numerous unexploited opportunities for clinicians, including doctors, nurses and other healthcare staff involved in patient care, to become involved in injury prevention.
- Trauma care – whether in the form of the initial response of the emergency services, first aid or subsequent treatment – is a form of tertiary prevention of injury.

Chapter 9. Changing patterns of health and disease

- Over the last century or so, there have been major improvements in global health.

- Most health variation between populations is likely to be due to environmental rather than genetic factors.
- Poverty remains the single most important underlying determinant of illness and injury in a population.
- Injuries are likely to become more problematic, in terms of both incidence and severity, for the world in the future.
- Globalisation is a double-edged sword in terms of injury prevention.
- Climate change is occurring and has serious implications for injury prevention.
- Perceived public health priorities (obesity, social inequalities and the early years) are changing and will have an impact on injury risk.
- Children are likely to be injured in greater numbers as anti-obesity measures are implemented.
- A focus on injury prevention will resonate strongly with aspirations to reduce inequality.
- The growing early years movement is perhaps the most exciting development in the entire public health landscape.

Chapter 10. Injury prevention in a changing world

- There is a wide variation in injury mortality rates across the globe.
- Sweden represents the epitome of good child safety policy and effective implementation.
- More than 95% of all injury deaths in children are estimated to occur in low- or middle-income countries.
- The United Nations and related bodies (especially the World Health Organization) have generally been a force for good in promoting child safety.
- To avoid fragmentation, achieve a critical mass of expertise and encourage a multidisciplinary approach, dedicated injury prevention centres have been created in many countries.

Chapter 11. The growing role of knowledge in injury prevention

- A wide implementation gap remains even in the world's wealthiest countries.
- The Internet has created unprecedented opportunities for the general public to access quickly and easily numerous authoritative sources of information.
- Capacity-building through knowledge and skills development of the workforce is one of the cornerstones of a comprehensive approach to injury prevention.

Chapter 12. Ethical aspects of injury prevention

- The decision to prevent injury requires a posture of presumed beneficence that is predicated on the assumption that the intervention will actually work.
- The two most effective strategic approaches (environmental modification and enforcement of legislation) imply a major role for government that some people may find philosophically or politically problematic.

■ The allocation of resources to injury prevention usually involves the denial of those resources to other deserving causes.

■ Child injury prevention can generate tensions between methodological, ideological or attitudinal polarities – populations versus individuals, prevention versus cure, unintentional versus intentional injury, young versus old.

■ The adoption of an evidence-based approach, with its emphasis on data-driven policy and practice, and a prominent role for evaluation ('to determine the value of') can hardly be regarded as value-free.

■ It would be unreasonable to exempt either public health generally or injury prevention specifically from rigorous and systematic ethical scrutiny.

References

Alexandrescu, R., O'Brien, S. J. and Lecky, F. E. (2009) 'A review of injury epidemiology in the UK and Europe: some methodological considerations in constructing rates', *BMC Public Health*, Vol. 9, p. 226

Allen, G. and Smith, I. D. (2008) *Early Intervention: Good Parents, Great Kids, Better Citizens*, London: Centre for Social Justice

Anderson, R. and Moxham, T. (2009) *Preventing Unintentional Injuries in Children: Systematic Review to Provide an Overview of Published Economic Evaluations of Relevant Legislation, Regulations, Standards and/or their Enforcement and Promotion by Mass Media*, Exeter: PenTAG

Antonovsky, A. (1996) 'The salutogenic model as a theory to guide health promotion', *Health Promotion International*, Vol. 11, pp. 11–18

Arbor, L. (2008) 'The responsibility to protect as a duty of care in international law and practice', *Review of International Studies*, Vol. 34, pp. 445–58

Audit Commission/Healthcare Commission (2007) *Better Safe than Sorry. Preventing Unintentional Injury in Children*, London: Audit Commission

Baker, S. P., O'Neill, B., Ginsburg, M. J. and Li, G. (eds.) (1992) *The Injury Fact Book*, 2nd edn, New York: Oxford University Press

Ballasteros, M. F., Jackson, M. L. and Martin, M. W. (2005) 'Working towards the elimination of residential fire deaths: the Centers for Disease Control and Prevention's smoke alarm installations and fire safety (SAIFE) program', *Journal of Burn Care and Rehabilitation*, Vol. 26, pp. 434–9

Barlow, J. (2007) 'The Webster Stratton "Incredible Years" parent training programme reduces conduct problems in children', *Evidence Based Mental Health*, Vol. 10, p. 86

Beaglehole, R. and Bonita, R. (1997) *Public Health at the Crossroads: Achievements and Prospects*, Cambridge: Cambridge University Press

Bellagio Study Group on Child Survival. (2003) 'How many child deaths can we prevent this year?', *Lancet*, Vol. 362, pp. 65–71

Ben-Shlomo, Y. and Kuh, D. (2002) 'A life course approach to chronic disease epidemiology: conceptual models, empirical challenges and interdisciplinary perspectives', *International Journal of Epidemiology*, Vol. 31, pp. 285–93.

Bergman, A. B. and Rivara, F. P. (1991) 'Sweden's experience in reducing childhood injuries', *Pediatrics*, Vol. 88, pp. 69–74

British Medical Association. (2001) *Injury Prevention*, London: BMA

Brown, C. E., Chishti, P. and Stone, D. H. (2005) 'Measuring socio-economic inequalities in the presentation of injuries to a paediatric A&E department: the importance of an epidemiological approach', *Public Health*, Vol. 119, pp. 721–5

Brussoni, M., Towner, E. and Hayes, M. (2006) 'Evidence into practice: combining the art and science of injury prevention', *Injury Prevention*, Vol. 12, pp. 373–7

Carnegie Commission on Preventing Deadly Conflict. (1997) *Final Report*, New York: Carnegie Corporation of New York

Cassell, E., Ashby, K., Guy, J. and Congiu, M. (2007) *Evaluation of the Effectiveness of the 2005 Victorian Personal Flotation Device (PFD) Wear Regulations: A Pre- and Post-observational Study.* Prepared for Marine Safety Victoria, Melbourne: Monash University Accident Research Centre

Cawson, P., Wattam, C., Brooker, S. and Kelly, G. (2000) *Child Maltreatment in the United Kingdom: A Study of the Prevalence of Child Abuse and Neglect*, London: NSPCC

Chalmers, D. J., Marshall, S.W., Langley, J. D., Evans, M. J., Brunton, C. R., Kelly, A. M., *et al.* (1996) 'Height and surfacing as risk factors for injury in falls from playground equipment: a case-control study', *Injury Prevention*, Vol. 2, pp. 98–104

References

Christie, N. (1995) *Social, Economic and Environmental Factors in Child Pedestrian Accidents: A Research Overview*. Report No. 16, Wokingham, Berkshire: Transport Research Laboratory

Christoffel, T. and Gallagher, S. S. (2006) *Injury Prevention and Public Health*, 2nd edn, Sudbury, MA: Jones & Bartlett

Committee on Trauma Research, Institute of Medicine, National Research Council (1985) *Injury in America: A Continuing Public Health Problem*, Washington, DC: Committee on Trauma Research/Institute of Medicine/National Research Council

Conners, G. P., Veenema, T. G., Kavanagh, C. A., Ricci, J. and Callahan, C. M. (2002) 'Still falling: a community-wide infant walker injury prevention initiative', *Patient Education and Counselling*, Vol. 46, pp. 169–73

Creighton, S. and Russell, N. (1995) *Voices from Childhood: A Survey of Childhood Experiences and Attitudes to Childrearing Among Adults in the United Kingdom*,
London: NSPCC

Crume, T. L., DiGuisepp, C., Byers, T., Sirotnak, A. P. and Garrett, C. J. (2002) 'Underascertainment of child maltreatment fatalities by death certificates, 1990–1998', *Pediatrics*, Vol. 110, pp. e18

Cryer, C. (2006) 'Severity of injury measures and descriptive epidemiology', *Injury Prevention*, Vol. 12, pp. 67–8

Dahlberg, L. L. and Krug, E. G. (2002) 'Violence – a global public health problem', in Krug, E., Dahlberg, L. L., Mercy, J. A., Zwi, A. B. and Lozano, R. (eds) *World Report on Violence and Health*, Geneva: World Health Organization, pp. 1–56

Dahlgren, G. and Whitehead, M. (1991) *Policies and Strategies to Promote Social Equity in Health*, Stockholm: Institute of Futures Studies

Davis, R. and Pless, I. B. (2001) 'BMJ bans "accidents"', *British Medical Journal*, Vol. 322, pp. 1320–1

Department for Children, Schools and Families (2008) *The Staying Safe Action Plan*, Nottingham: DCSF

Department of Health (2002) *Preventing Accidental Injury – Priorities for Action*. Report to the Chief Medical Officer from the Accidental Injury Task Force, London: The Stationery Office

Department of Health and Human Services. (2001) *National Strategy for Suicide Prevention: Goals and Objectives*. Rockville, MD: DHHS Public Health Service

Donabedian, A. (2003) *An Introduction to Quality Assurance in Health Care*, New York: Oxford University Press

Duperrex, O., Bunn, F. and Roberts, I. (2002) 'Safety education of pedestrians for injury prevention: a systematic review of randomised controlled trials', *British Medical Journal*, Vol. 324, p. 1129–34

Eraut, M. (1994) *Developing Professional Knowledge and Competence*, London: Falmer Press

Esselman, P. C. (2007) 'Burn rehabilitation: an overview', *Archives of Physical and Medical Rehabilitation*, Vol. 88 (Suppl. 2), pp. S3–6

Evans, R. G. and Stoddart, G. L. (1990) 'Producing health, consuming health care', *Social Science and Medicine*, 31, pp. 1347–63

Feldman, K. W., Schaller, R. T., Feldman, J. A. and McMillon, M. (1998) '*Tap water scald burns in children*', *Injury Prevention*, Vol. 4, pp. 238–42

Felitti, V. J., Anda, R. F., Nordenberg, D., Williamson, D. F., Spitz, A. M., Edwards, V., *et al.* (1998) 'Relationship of childhood abuse and household dysfunction to many of the leading causes of death in adults. The Adverse Childhood Experiences (ACE) Study', *American Journal of Preventive Medicine*, Vol. 14, pp. 245–58

Fenner, P. J., Harrison, S. L., Williamson, J. A. and Williamson, B. D. (1995) 'Success of surf lifesaving resuscitations in Queensland, 1973–1992', *Medical Journal of Australia*, Vol. 163, pp. 580–3

Fingerhut, L. A. (2004) 'International collaborative effort on injury statistics: 10-year review', *Injury Prevention*, Vol. 10, pp. 264–7

Flanagan, R., Rooney, C. and Griffiths, C. (2005) 'Fatal poisoning in childhood, England and Wales, 1968–2000', *Forensic Science International*, Vol. 148, pp. 121–9

Geddes, R., Haw, S. and Frank, J. (2010) *Interventions for Promoting Early Child Development for Health. An Environmental Scan with Special Reference to Scotland*, Edinburgh: Scottish Collaboration for Public Health Research and Policy

Gillon, R. (1994) 'Medical ethics: four principles plus attention to scope', *British Medical Journal*, Vol. 309, pp. 184–8

Girasek, D. C. (1999) 'How members of the public interpret the word accident', *Injury Prevention*, Vol. 5, pp. 19–25

Gordon, J. (1949) 'The epidemiology of accidents', *American Journal of Public Health*, Vol. 39, pp. 504–15

Graham, G., Glaister, S. and Anderson, R. (2005) 'The effects of area deprivation on the incidence of child and adult pedestrian casualties in England', *Accident Analysis and Prevention*, Vol. 37, pp. 125–35

Grundy, C., Steinbach, R., Edwards, P., Green, J., Armstrong, B. and Wilkinson, P. (2009) 'Effect of 20 mph traffic speed zones on road injuries in London, 1986–2006: controlled interrupted time series analysis', *British Medical Journal*, Vol. 339, p. b4469

Guo, B. and Harstall, C. (2004) *For Which Strategies of Suicide Prevention Is There Evidence of Effectiveness?*, Copenhagen: WHO Regional Office for Europe

Haddon, W. (1999) 'The changing approach to the epidemiology, prevention, and amelioration of trauma: the transition to approaches etiologically rather than descriptively based', *Injury Prevention*, Vol. 5, pp. 231–5

Han, R. K., Ungar, W. J. and Macarthur, C. (2007) 'Cost-effectiveness analysis of a proposed public health legislative/educational strategy to reduce tap water scald injuries in children', *Injury Prevention*, Vol. 13, pp. 248–53

Hawton, K. and Harris, L. (2008) 'How often does deliberate self-harm occur relative to each suicide? A study of variations by gender and age', *Suicide and Life-threatening Behavior*, Vol. 38, pp. 650–60

Hawton, K., Rodham, K., Evans, E. and Weatherall, R. (2002) 'Deliberate self harm in adolescents: self report survey in schools in England', *British Medical Journal*, Vol. 325, pp. 1207–11

Hemenway, D. (2009) *While We Were Sleeping. Success Stories in Injury and Violence Prevention*, Berkeley: University of California Press

Heptinstall, E. (1996) *Healing the Hidden Hurt*, London: Child Accident Prevention Trust

Holder, Y., Peden, M., Krug, E., Lund, J., Gururaj, G. and Kobusingye, O. (eds) (2001) *Injury Surveillance Guidelines*, Geneva: World Health Organization

Horrocks, A. R., Nazare, S. and Kandola, B. (2004) 'The particular flammability hazards of nightwear', *Fire Safety Journal*, Vol. 39, pp. 259–76

Hosking, G. D. C. and Walsh, I. R. (2005) *The WAVE Report 2005: Violence and what to do about it*, Croydon: WAVE Trust.

Hynd, D., Cuerden, R., Reid, S. and Adams, S. (2009) *The Potential for Cycle Helmets to Prevent Injury – a Review of the Evidence*, Wokingham, Berkshire: Transport Research Laboratory

Intergovernmental Panel on Climate Change; Pachauri, R. K. and Reisinger, A (eds.) (2007) *Climate Change 2007: Synthesis Report. Contribution of Working Groups I, II and III to the Fourth Assessment Report of the Intergovernmental Panel on Climate Change*, Geneva: IPCC

Jackson, R. H. (1995) 'The history of childhood accident and injury prevention in England: background to the foundation of the Child Accident Prevention Trust', *Injury Prevention*, Vol. 1, pp. 4–6

Jacobs, G., Thomas, A. A. and Astrop, A. (2000) *Estimating Global Road Fatalities*, Wokingham, Berkshire: Transport Research Laboratory

James-Ellison, M., Barnes, P., Maddocks, A., Wareham, K., Drew, P., Dickson, W., *et al.* (2009) 'Social health outcomes following thermal injuries: a retrospective matched cohort study', *Archives of Disease in Childhood*, Vol. 94, pp. 663–7

Jansson, B., Ponce de Leon, A., Ahmed, N. and Jansson, V. (2006) 'Why does Sweden have the lowest child injury mortality in the world?', *Journal of Public Health Policy*, Vol. 27, pp. 146–65

Jeffrey, S., Stone, D. H., Blamey, A., Clark, D., Cooper, C., Dickson, K., *et al.* (2009) 'An evaluation of police reporting of road casualties', *Injury Prevention*, Vol. 15, pp. 13–18

Johnston, B. (2010) 'Road traffic injury prevention', *Injury Prevention*, Vol. 16, p. 1

Karkhaneh, M., Kalenga, J. C., Hagel, B. E. and Rowe, B. H. (2006) 'Effectiveness of bicycle helmet legislation to increase helmet use: a systematic review', *Injury Prevention*, Vol. 12, pp. 76–82

Kass, N. (2004) 'Public health ethics. From foundations and frameworks to justice and global public health', *Journal of Law, Medicine, and Ethics*, Vol. 32, pp. 232–42

References

Kelly, M. P., Chambers, J., Huntley, J. and Millward, L. (2004) *Evidence Into Practice: Method 1 for the Production of Effective Action Briefings and Related Materials*, London: Health Development Agency

Kemp, A. M. and Sibert, J. R. (1991) 'Outcomes in children who nearly drown: a British Isles study', *British Medical Journal*, Vol. 302, pp. 931–3

Kempe, C. H., Silverman, F. N., Steele, B. F., Droegmuller, W. and Silver, H. K. (1962) 'The battered-child syndrome', *Journal of the American Medical Association*, Vol. 181, pp. 17–24

Kendrick, D., Barlow, J., Hampshire, A., Polnay, L. and Stewart-Brown, S. (2007) 'Parenting interventions for the prevention of unintentional injuries in childhood', *Cochrane Database of Systematic Reviews*, Issue 4, Art. No. CD006020

Kendrick, D., Mulvaney, C. and Watson, M. (2009) 'Does targeting injury prevention towards families in disadvantaged areas reduce inequalities in safety practice?', *Health Education Research*, Vol. 1, pp. 32–41

Khambalia, A., Joshi, P., Brussoni, M., Raina, P., Morrongiello, B. and Macarthur, C. (2006) 'Risk factors for unintentional injuries due to falls in children aged 0–6 years: a systematic review', *Injury Prevention*, Vol. 12, pp. 378–81

Krug, E., Dahlberg, L. L., Mercy, J. A., Zwi, A. B. and Lozano, R. (eds) (2002) *World Report on Violence and Health*, Geneva: World Health Organization

Laforest, S., Robitaille, Y., Lesage, D. and Dorval, D. (2001) 'Surface characteristics, equipment height, and the occurrence and severity of playground injuries', *Injury Prevention*, Vol. 7, pp. 35–40

Lalonde, M. (1974) *A New Perspective on the Health of Canadians*, Ottawa: Government of Canada

Lazenbatt, A. (2010) 'The impact of abuse and neglect on the health and mental health of children and young people' (online). Available from URL: www.nspcc.org.uk/Inform/research/briefings/impact_of_abuse_on_health_pdf_wdf73369.pdf (accessed 7 February 2011)

Louwers, E. C. F. M., Affourtit, M. J., Moll, H. A., de Koning, H. J. and Korfage, I. J. (2010) 'Screening for child abuse at emergency departments: a systematic review', *Archives of Disease in Childhood*, Vol. 95, pp. 214–18

Lyons, R. A., Jones, S., Kemp, A., Shepherd, J., Richmond, P., Bartlett, C., *et al.* (2002) 'Development and use of a population based surveillance system: the All Wales Injury Surveillance System (AWISS)', *Injury Prevention*, Vol. 8, pp. 83–6

Lyons, R. A., Ward, H., Brunt, H., Macey, S., Thoreau, R., Bodger, O. G., *et al.* (2008) 'Using multiple datasets to understand trends in serious road casualties', *Accident Analysis and Prevention*, Vol. 40, pp. 1406–10

MacInnes, K. and Stone, D. H. (2008) 'Stages of development and injury: an epidemiological survey of young children presenting to an emergency department', *BMC Public Health*, Vol. **8**, p. 120

Mackay, M., Vincenten, J., Brussoni, M. and Towner, L. (2006) *Child Safety Good Practice Guide: Good Investments in Unintentional Child Injury Prevention and Safety Promotion*, Amsterdam: European Child Safety Alliance/EuroSafe

MacKenzie, E. J., Steinwachs, D. M. and Shankar, B. (1989) 'Classifying trauma severity based on hospital discharge diagnoses. Validation of an ICD-9-CM to AIS-85 conversion table', *Medical Care*, Vol. 27, pp. 412–22

McLoughlin, E., Clarke, N., Stahl, K. and Crawford, J. D. (1977) 'One pediatric burn unit's experience with sleepwear-related injuries', *Pediatrics*, Vol. 60, pp. 405–9

McVeigh, C., Hughes, K., Bellis, M. A., Reed, E., Ashton, J. R. and Syed, Q. (2005) *Violent Britain: People, Prevention and Public Health*, Liverpool: John Moores University

Madge, N., Hewitt, A., Hawton, K., Wilde, E. J., Corcoran, P., Fekete, S., *et al.* (2008) 'Deliberate self-harm within an international community sample of young people: comparative findings from the Child & Adolescent Self-harm in Europe (CASE) Study', *Journal of Child Psychology and Psychiatry*, Vol. 49, pp. 667–77

Mallonee, S. (2000) 'Evaluating injury prevention programs: the Oklahoma City Smoke Alarm Project', *Future Child*, Vol. 10, pp. 164–74

Mallonee, S., Fowler, C. and Istre, G. R. (2006) 'Bridging the gap between research and practice: a continuing challenge', *Injury Prevention*, Vol. 12, pp. 357–9

Mann, J. J., Apter, A., Bertolote, J., Beautrais, A., Currier, D., Haas, A., *et al.* (2005) 'Suicide prevention strategies: a systematic review', *Journal of the American Medical Association*, Vol. 294, pp. 2064–74

References

Manolios, N. and Mackie, I. (1988) 'Drowning and near-drowning on Australian beaches patrolled by life-savers: a 10-year study, 1973–1983', *Medical Journal of Australia*, Vol. 148, pp. 170–1

Mathers, C. and Loncar, D. (2005) *Updated Projections of Global Mortality and Burden of Disease, 2002–2030: Data Sources, Methods and Results*, Geneva: World Health Organization

Miller, T. R. and Hendrie, D. (2005) 'How should government spend the drug prevention dollar? A buyer's guide', in Stockwell, T., Gruenwald, P. J., Toumbourou, J. W. and Loxley, W. (eds) *Preventing Harmful Substance Use: The Evidence Base for Policy and Practice*, Hoboken, NJ: John Wiley & Sons, pp. 415–31

Morency, P. and Cloutier, M.-S. (2006) 'From targeted "black spots" to area-wide pedestrian safety', *Injury Prevention*, Vol. 12, pp. 360–4

Morris, G. P., Beck, S. A., Hanlon, P. and Robertson, R. (2006) 'Getting strategic about the environment and health', *Public Health*, Vol. 120, pp. 889–903

Morrison, A. and Stone, D. H. (1998) 'Injury surveillance in accident and emergency departments: to sample or not to sample?', *Injury Prevention*, Vol. 4, pp. 50–3

Murray, C. J. L. and Lopez, A. D. (1997a) 'Alternative projections of mortality and disability by cause 1990–2020: Global Burden of Disease Study', *Lancet*, Vol. 349, pp. 1498–504

Murray, C. J. L. and Lopez, A. D. (1997b) 'Mortality by cause for eight regions of the world: Global Burden of Disease Study', *Lancet*, Vol. 349, pp. 1269–76

Nader, R. (1965) *Unsafe at Any Speed*, New York: Grossman

National Audit Office (2010) *Major Trauma Care in England*, London: The Stationery Office

National Institute for Health and Clinical Excellence. (2009) *Preventing Unintentional Injuries in Children: Systematic Review to Provide an Overview of Published Economic Evaluations of Relevant Legislation, Regulations, Standards, and/or their Enforcement and Promotion by Mass Media*. Final Report, London: NICE

National Institute for Health and Clinical Excellence. (2010) 'Injuries, accidents and wounds' (online). Available from URL: http://guidance.nice.org.uk/Topic/InjuriesAccidentsWounds (accessed 7 February 2011)

Nicholl, J. P. (2006) 'Health research funding', *British Medical Journal*, Vol. 332, p. 1510

Olds, D. L. and Henderson, C. R. (1986) 'Preventing child abuse and neglect; a randomised trial of nurse home visitation', *Pediatrics*, Vol. 78, pp. 65–78

Olds, D. L., Robinson, J., Pettitt, L., Luckey, D. W., Holmberg, J., Ng, R. K., *et al.* (2004) 'Effects of home visits by paraprofessionals and by nurses: age 4 follow up results of a randomised trial', *Pediatrics*, Vol. 114, pp. 1560–8

Osler, T., Rutledge, R., Deis, J. and Bedrick, E. (1996) 'An International Classification of Disease-9 based injury severity score', *Journal of Trauma*, Vol. 41, pp. 380–8

Pearson, J., Jeffrey, S. and Stone, D. H. (2009) 'Varying gender pattern of childhood injury mortality over time in Scotland', *Archives of Disease in Childhood*, Vol. 94, pp. 524–30

Peden, M., Scurfield, R., Sleet, D., Mohan, D., Hyder, A. A., Jarawan, E., *et al.* (2004) *World Report on Road Traffic Injury Prevention*, Geneva: World Health Organization

Peden, M., Oyegbite, K., Ozanne-Smith, J., Hyder, A. A., Branche, C., Rahman, A. K. M. F., *et al.* (eds) (2008) *World Report on Child Injury Prevention*, Geneva: World Health Organization/UNICEF

Petridou, E., Simou, E., Skondras, C., Pistevos, G., Lagos, P. and Papoutsakis, G. (1996) 'Hazards of baby walkers in a European context', *Injury Prevention*, Vol. 2, pp. 118–20

Petridou, E. T., Kyllekidis, S., Jeffrey, S., Chishti, P., Dessypris, N. and Stone, D. H. (2007) 'Unintentional injury mortality in the European Union: how many more lives could be saved?', *Scandinavian Journal of Public Health*, Vol. 35, pp. 278–87

Pless, I. B. (2006) 'A brief history of injury and accident prevention publications', *Injury Prevention*, Vol. 12, pp. 65–6

Pless, I. B. and Hagel, B. E. (2005) 'Injury prevention: a glossary of terms', *Journal of Epidemiology and Community Health*, Vol. 59, pp. 182–5

Prinz, R. J., Sanders, M. R., Shapiro, C. J., Whitaker, D. J. and Lutzker, J. R. (2009) 'Population-based prevention of child maltreatment: the U.S. Triple P system population trial', *Prevention Science*, Vol. 10, pp. 1–12

References

Rivara, C. F. (1998) 'Hot water scald burns in children', *Paediatrics*, Vol. 102, pp. 256–8

Rivara, F. P. and Grossman, D. C. (1996) 'Prevention of traumatic deaths to children in the United States: how far have we come and where do we need to go?', *Pediatrics*, Vol. 97, pp. 791–7

Roberts, H., Smith, S. J. and Bryce, C. (1995) *Children at Risk? Safety as a Social Value*, Buckingham: Open University Press

Roberts, I. and Hillman, M. (2009) 'Climate change: the implications for injury control and health promotion', *Injury Prevention*, Vol. 11, pp. 326–9

Roberts, I., Campbell, F., Hollis, S. and Yates, D. (1996) 'Reducing accident death rates in children and young adults: the contribution of hospital care', *British Medical Journal*, Vol. 313, pp. 1239–41

Robinson, D. L. (2006) 'No clear evidence from countries that have enforced the wearing of helmets', *British Medical Journal*, Vol. 332, pp. 722–5

Rose, G. (1981) 'Strategy of prevention: lessons from cardiovascular disease', *British Medical Journal*, Vol. 282, pp. 1847–51

Rosenberg, M. L. and Mercy, J. A. (1991) 'Assaultive violence', in Rosenberg, M. L. and Fenley, M. A. (eds) *Violence in America: A Public Health Approach*. New York: Oxford University Press, pp. 14–50

Royal Society for the Prevention of Accidents/Child Accident Prevention Trust. (2007) *Child Safety Strategy. Preventing Unintentional Injuries to Children and Young People in Scotland*, Edinburgh: RoSPA

Runyan, C. W. (1998) 'Using the Haddon matrix: introducing the third dimension', *Injury Prevention*, Vol. 4, pp. 302–7

Runyan, C. W., Bangdiwala, S. I., Linzer, M. A., Sacks, J. J. and Butts, J. (1992) '*Risk factors for fatal residential fires*', *New England Journal of Medicine*, Vol. *327, pp. 859–63*

Sackett, D. L. and Straus, S. E. (1998) 'Finding and applying evidence during clinical rounds: the "evidence cart"', *Journal of the American Medical Association*, Vol. 280, pp. 1336–8

Sackett, D., Straus, S. E., Richardson, W. S., Rosenberg, W. and Haynes, R. B. (2000) *Evidence-Based Medicine: How to Practice and Teach EBM*, 2nd edn, London: Churchill Livingstone

Sanders, M. R. (2008) 'Triple P-Positive Parenting Program as a public health approach to strengthening parenting', *Journal of Family Psychology*, Vol. 22, pp. 506–17

Schopper, D., Lormand, J.-D. and Waxweiler, R. (eds) (2006) *Developing Policies to Prevent Injuries and Violence: Guidelines for Policy-makers and Planners*, Geneva: World Health Organization

Scriven, M. (1998) 'Minimalist theory of evaluation: the least theory that practice requires', *American Journal of Evaluation*, Vol. 19, pp. 57–70

Sethi, D., Racioppi, F., Baumgarten, I. and Vida P. (2005) *Injuries and Violence in Europe. Why They Matter and What Can Be Done*, Copenhagen: WHO Regional Office for Europe

Sethi, D., Towner, E., Vincenten, J., Segui-Gomez, M. and Racioppi, F. (2008) *European Report on Child Injury Prevention*, Copenhagen: World Health Organization

Sherker, S., Ozanne-Smith, J., Rechnitzer, G. and Grzebieta, R. (2005) 'Out on a limb: risk factors for arm fracture in playground equipment falls', *Injury Prevention*, Vol. 11, pp. 120–4

Shipton, D. and Stone, D. H. (2008) '*The Yorkhill CHIRPP story: a qualitative evaluation of 10 years of injury surveillance at a Scottish children's hospital*', *Injury Prevention*, Vol. 14, pp. 245–9

Sidel, V. W. and Levy, B. S. (2009) 'Collective violence: war', in Detels, R., Beaglehole, R., Lansang, M. A. and Gulliford, M. (eds) *Oxford Textbook of Public Health*, 5th edn, Vol 3, Oxford: Oxford University Press, pp. 1367–75

Sivarajasingam, V., Shepherd, J. P., Matthews, K. and Jones, S. (2003) 'Violence-related injury data in England and Wales. An alternative data source on violence', *British Journal of Criminology*, Vol. 43, pp. 223–7

Sminkey, L. A. (2006) 'Finding a common vision for injury prevention, *Injury Prevention*, Vol. 12, p. 171

Smith, L., Smith, C. and Ray, D. (1991) *Lighters and Matches: An Assessment of Risk Associated with Household Ownership and Use*, Washington, DC: United States Consumer Product Safety Commission

Smith, L. E., Greene, M. A. and Singh, H. A. (2002) 'Study of the effectiveness of the US safety standard for child-resistant cigarette lighters', *Injury Prevention*, Vol. 8, pp. 192–6

Spiegel, C. N. and Lindaman, F. C. (1977) 'Children Can't Fly: a program to prevent childhood morbidity and mortality from window falls', *American Journal of Public Health*, Vol. 61, pp. 90–6

Stone, D. H. (1996) 'Research on injury prevention: time for an international agenda?', *Journal of Epidemiology and Community Health*, Vol. 50, pp. 127–30

Stone, D. H. and Pearson, J. (2009) 'Unintentional injury prevention: what can paediatricians do?', *Archives of Disease in Childhood Education and Practice Edition*, Vol. 94, pp. 102–7

Stone, D. H., Morrison, A. and Ohn, T. T. (1998) 'Developing injury surveillance in accident and emergency departments', *Archives of Disease in Childhood*, Vol. 78, pp. 108–10

Stone, D. H., Morrison, A. and Smith, G. S. (1999) 'Emergency department injury surveillance systems: the best use of limited resources?', *Injury Prevention*, Vol. 5, pp. 166–7

Stone, D. H., Jeffrey, S., Dessypris, N., Kyllekidis, P., Chishti, P., Papdopoulos, F. C., *et al.* (2006) 'Intentional injury mortality in the European Union: how many more lives could be saved?', *Injury Prevention*, Vol. 12, pp. 327–32

Taft, C., Paul, H., Consunji, R. and Miller, T. (2002) *Childhood Unintentional Injury Worldwide: Meeting the Challenge*, Washington, DC: SAFE KIDS Worldwide

Thomas, J., Kavanagh, J., Tucker, H., Burchett, H., Tripney, J. and Oakley, A. (2007) *Accidental Injury, Risk Taking Behaviour and the Social Circumstances in Which Young People (aged 12–24) Live: A Systematic Review*, London: EPPI-Centre Institute of Education

Thompson, D. C. and Rivara, F. P. (2000) 'Pool fencing for preventing drowning in children', *Cochrane Database of Systematic Reviews*, Issue 2, Art. No. CD001047.

Thompson, D. C., Rivara, F. P. and Thompson, R. (2005) 'Helmets for preventing head and facial injuries in bicyclists', *Cochrane Database of Systematic Reviews*, Issue 4, Art. No. CD001855

Thomson, J. K. and Whelan, K. M. (1997) *A Community Approach to Road Safety Education Using Practical Training Methods*. Road Safety Research Report No. 3, London: Department for Transport

Thygerson, A. L., Thygerson, S.M. and Thygerson, J. S. (2008) *Injury Prevention. Competencies for Unintentional Injury Prevention Professionals*, 3rd edn, Sudbury, MA: Jones & Bartlett

Towner, E. and Towner, J. (2001) *Study of Effective Measures in Reducing Childhood Deaths and Serious Injuries in 29 OECD Countries. A League Table of Child Deaths by Injury in Rich Nations. Innocenti Report Card No. 2*, Florence: UNICEF Innocenti Research Centre

Towner, E. and Ward, H. (1998) 'Prevention of injuries to children and young people: the way ahead for the UK', *Injury Prevention*, Vol. **4**, pp. S17–25

Tremblay, R. E. (2006) 'Prevention of youth violence: why not start at the beginning?', *Journal of Abnormal Child Psychology*, Vol. 34, pp. 481–7

Tudor Hart, J. (1971) 'The inverse care law', *Lancet*, Vol. 1, pp. 405–12

Turner, C., McClure, R., Nixon, J. and Spinks, A. (2004). 'Community-based programmes to prevent pedestrian injuries in children 0–14 years: a systematic review'. *Injury Control and Safety Promotion*, Vol. 11, pp. 231–7

Turvill, J. L., Burroughs, A. K. and Moore, K. P. (2000) 'Change in occurrence of paracetamol overdose in UK after introduction of blister packs', *Lancet*, Vol. 355, pp. 2048–9

Unites States Coast Guard. (2010) *Recreational Boating Statistics 2009*, Washington, DC: US Department of Homeland Security

Valent, F., Little, D., Bertollini, R., Nemer, L. E., Barbone, F. and Tamburlini, G. (2004) 'Burden of disease attributable to selected environmental factors and injury among children and adolescents in Europe', *Lancet*, Vol. 363, pp. 2032–9

Villavecas, A., Kammeyer, J. A. and Bencevic, H. (2005) 'Injury prevention education in medical schools: an international survey of medical students', *Injury Prevention*, Vol. 11, pp. 343–7

Villaveces, A., Christiansen, A. and Hargartern, S. W. (2010) 'Developing a global research agenda on violence and injury prevention: a modest proposal', *Injury Prevention*, Vol. 16, pp. 190–3

Vyrostek, S. B., Annest, J. L. and Ryan, G. W. (2004) 'Surveillance for fatal and nonfatal injuries – United States, 2001', *Morbidity and Mortality Weekly Report*, Vol. 53, 1–57

Walton, W. W. (1982) 'An evaluation of the Poison Prevention Packaging Act', *Paediatrics*, Vol. 69, pp. 363–70

Wanless, D. (2004) *Securing Good Health for the Whole Population: Final Report*, London: HM Treasury

References

Ward, H. and Christie, N. (2000) *Strategic Review of Research Priorities for Accidental Injury*, London: University College London/Transport Research Laboratory

Watson, M., Kendrick, D., Coupland, C., Woods, A., Futer, D. and Robinson, J. (2005) 'Providing child safety equipment to prevent injuries: randomised controlled trial', *British Medical Journal*, Vol. 330, p. 178

White, D., Raeside, R. and Barker, D. (2000) *Road Accidents and Children Living in Disadvantaged Areas: A Literature Review*, Edinburgh: Scottish Executive Central Research Unit

Wikler, D. I. (1978) 'Coercive measures in health promotion: can they be justified?', *Health Education Monographs*, Vol. 6, pp. 223–41

Wilkinson, R. G. (1992) 'Income distribution and life expectancy', *British Medical Journal*, Vol. 304, pp. 165–8

Wilson, J. M. G. and Jungner, G. (1968) *Principles and Practice of Screening for Disease*. Public Health Paper No. 34, Geneva: World Health Organization

World Health Organization. (2003) *Guidelines for Safe Recreational Water Environments, Vol 1. Coastal and Fresh Waters*. Geneva: WHO

World Health Organization. (2006) *Helmets: A Road Safety Manual for Decision-makers and Practitioners*, Geneva: WHO

World Health Organization/John Moores University. (2009) *Violence Prevention – the Evidence*, Geneva: WHO

Wright, C. M., Jeffrey, S., Ross, M. K., Wallis, L. and Wood, R. (2009) 'Targeting health visitor care: lessons from Starting Well', *Archives of Disease in Childhood*, Vol. **94**, pp. 23–7

Zolotor, A. J., Theodore, A. D., Change, J. J., Berkoff, M. C. and Runyan, D. K. (2008) 'Speak softly and forget the stick', *American Journal of Preventive Medicine*, Vol. 35, pp. 364–9

Some web-based sources of further information

American Academic of Pediatrics: www.aap.org/family/tippmain.htm

Bicycle Helmet Initiative Trust (UK): www.bhit.org/

Centers for disease Control and Prevention (USA): www.cdc.gov/ncipc/factsheets/children.htm

Child Accident Prevention Trust (UK): www.capt.org.uk/

EuroSafe (European Child Safety Alliance): www.eurosafe.eu.com/csi/eurosafe.nsf/html/homepage/$file/index.htm

Injury Observatory for Britain and Ireland: www.injuryobservatory.net/

Injury Prevention journal: http://injuryprevention.bmj.com/

National Institute for Health and Clinical Excellence (UK): http://guidance.nice.org.uk/Topic/InjuriesAccidentsWounds

Royal Society for the Prevention of Accidents (UK): www.rospa.com/childsafety/

World Health Organization Helmet Initiative: www.whohelmets.org/

World Health Organization Violence and Injury Prevention and Disability: www.who.int/violence_injury_prevention/child/en/

Index

Note: page numbers in **bold** refer to glossary items; those in *italics* to figures or tables